DAVID COHEN

Soviet Psychiatry

PALADIN
GRAFTON BOOKS
A Division of the Collins Publishing Group

LONDON GLASGOW
TORONTO SYDNEY AUCKLAND

Paladin
Grafton Books
A Division of the Collins Publishing Group
8 Grafton Street, London W1X 3LA

A Paladin Paperback Original 1989

A CIP catalogue record for this book
is available from the British Library

ISBN 0-586-08934-9

Printed and bound in Great Britain by
Collins, Glasgow

Set in Times

Contents

Preface

There are some stories it seems impossible to get – access to Soviet psychiatric hospitals has long seemed one of those eternally elusive ones.

In 1987, the day after the transmission of *Forgotten Millions*, a film which looked at mental health care in Japan, America, Egypt and India, I received a telephone call from Dr Julian Goodburn and Trish Thomas. They said they thought it would be possible to arrange a similar film about the USSR. We met the week after and, though I was sceptical, I thought the opportunity far too good to miss. We sent letters and telexes to Moscow. For months, there was no progress. Goodburn and Thomas had good contacts with Novosti, the Soviet press agency, but clearly the issue was too sensitive.

Then, Goodburn and Thomas visited the USSR themselves in February 1988. After that, we managed to interest Channel 4, and the three of us went back in September 1988 to negotiate with the Soviet authorities. I know that there are many emphases in the book that both Goodburn and Thomas won't agree with, but I want to record my thanks to them. Without their enthusiasm and belief that it could happen, neither the film *Dispatches: Gorbachev's Asylums* nor this book would have materialized.

There are many others who made the project possible. David Lloyd, Senior Commissioning Editor at Channel 4, and Karen Brown, Assistant Commissioning Editor for current affairs, were keen on the project from the start and very supportive throughout the production.

Novosti assigned us two of their staff – Eleonora Gorbunova, their health correspondent, and Yelena Ushina – who helped a great deal in arranging access for us. Yelena also undertook much of the translating. Two of the chief functionaries of Novosti in Moscow, A. Bogamolov and Anatoly Smirnoff, the deputy head of the video department, were also very helpful, as was Viktor Orlik, the bureau head in London. I also want to thank Daphne Skillen, the researcher on the film, and Jan Euden.

This is not, however, the book of the film. *Dispatches* ran for forty minutes, and I gathered far more material than could be used in the film. Many commentators on Soviet affairs believe that psychiatry is one area in which perestroika and glasnost face the greatest problems. What follows should help clarify this important, and perplexing, issue.

1

The Dissident and the Woman Who Cannot Lose Her Husband

In 1983, the Soviet Association of Neuropathologists and Psychiatrists resigned from the World Psychiatric Association. It did so to avoid an angry debate at the association's Vienna Congress on the political abuse of psychiatry. The debate might well have demanded an inquiry into Soviet practices or even the expulsion of the Soviet Association. The Soviets denied they had too much to hide. Rather, they claimed they were resigning because they didn't want grubby politics to sully the pure science of psychiatry. Slandering their hospitals was part of the cold war. Few in the West took their reasons seriously. Psychiatrists don't like doubting their colleagues. It had taken twelve years of lobbying, and much hard evidence, to persuade the World Psychiatric Association that it had to act.

The accusations of political abuse aroused passion in the West and bitterness in the East. Soviet psychiatry retreated behind its own Iron Curtain. From 1970 on, when the dissident issue first arose, it was hard for Western doctors, and almost impossible for Western journalists, to visit Soviet hospitals. They became 'no go areas'.

The Soviet Union now wants to rejoin the World Psychiatric Association. Its psychiatrists are under considerable pressure, since Gorbachev's new policies actively encourage openness and contact with foreigners. Giving me access to some of the most 'notorious' institutions like the Serbsky Institute and the Leningrad Special Hospital was clearly a political decision taken, I suspect, by the Ministry of Health. That Ministry now seems to be in total control of psychiatry. Till 1988, the Ministry of the Interior which runs the police and has close links with the KGB, supervised all top-security hospitals.

The Soviets want to show that their human rights record is

improving. It would be useful to trumpet that perestroika and glasnost extend even into these forbidden areas.

Soviet psychiatry lost a good deal by making itself inaccessible. First, it reinforced the suspicion that it had much to hide. Second, its relative isolation meant it didn't learn about many progressive ideas in the West. Very few Soviet psychiatrists travelled outside Eastern Europe. In addition, the West remained ignorant of positive developments in the USSR – and there have been some. Worst of all, one of the largest 'psychiatries' in the world stayed shrouded in secrecy. The Soviet Union has some 25,000 psychiatrists, more than any country other than the United States.

Arranging the access was not as difficult as I had expected. Clearly, the Ministry of Health felt that the time had come to change tack. However, they were wary and so was I. The Soviet news agency, Novosti, agreed to 'render assistance' to the film I was making for Channel 4. It assigned its health correspondent, Eleonora Gorbunova, and a bright young fixer, Yelena Ushina, to the project. Their task was to facilitate access. When it became obvious they could do that splendidly, I faced my first problem. How much should I trust them?

For my film to be effective, I had to talk to dissidents who had spent time in hospitals and, also, to human rights activists. It was crucial to report what they felt about the new liberal climate. I was not sure how Novosti would react if I asked them to arrange meetings with such people. I didn't want my marvellous contacts to dry up, so I told them nothing. Long years of denying access breeds such subterfuges.

Specifically, I wanted to interview Alexander Podrabinek who wrote *Punitive Medicine*. In it, he exposed the political abuse of psychiatry in the seventies and early eighties. He had been a key figure in the group that monitored Soviet psychiatry after the 1975 Helsinki accords. For his pains, he spent five years in prison and exile.

One evening, telling Eleonora and Yelena that we were going to the theatre, Daphne Skillen, the researcher on the film, and I took a taxi to an apartment house in central Moscow. For twenty minutes, we couldn't find the flat we had been directed to. The hallways were dark; we used a lighter to see where we were going. We didn't dare ask anyone the way. Eventually we found the door with the right number but nobody answered the bell.

I began to wonder if I was being paid back for my lack of trust.

Daphne said we should wait. About two minutes after we'd rung the bell, we heard noises. Someone asked who was there. Inside, they were just being careful. When the door was finally opened, I noticed it had three weighty locks. Podrabinek doesn't live in the flat himself but it is used to help produce a journal called *Express Khronika*. It has taken over from the samizdat *Chronicle of Current Events*, but now it's not illegal to publish it.

Podrabinek is a small man with a beard. After writing *Punitive Medicine*, he was not allowed to finish his medical studies. He is now free but still in some form of technical exile. He has to live outside Moscow and can only spend three days a week in the city. I hoped that Podrabinek would give me his assessment of the new mood in psychiatry and some recently introduced reforms. I also hoped through him to meet men and women who had recently been in special hospitals. That evening he introduced me to one such person but they were too frightened of the consequences to be interviewed on film. Podrabinek agreed to be interviewed and promised to do his best to find some willing interviewees.

I didn't tell Novosti we had seen him. As Eleonora and Yelena negotiated our way into many hospitals, I began to worry I was being unfair to them. They were behaving as good colleagues, not ideological minders. I decided to test the water.

The *Medical Gazette* is the Soviet Union's most popular medical newspaper. It sells 500,000 copies, mainly to doctors. Andrei Mann, a young journalist, is its deputy editor. He had written a number of critical articles on psychiatry. Daphne and I made direct contact with him and arranged to film an interview. We then told Novosti what we had done. They were not pleased. We had paid them to 'render assistance', they said, so it was up to them to make such contacts. Eleonora Gorbunova said tartly that Mann wasn't an expert on psychiatry so why interview him? Novosti made no attempt to stop the interview but Yelena sat in on it.

The tension caused by our direct approach to Mann made me certain I had been right to be discreet about Podrabinek. We arranged to film him on a Sunday. To Novosti we said we were going to see yet another play. We slipped out of the hotel around six o'clock with no shred of video equipment visible. The camera was split between two bags. I carried a small light in my pocket; Daphne had the Betacam tapes in her handbag. We took a taxi back to the flat.

Podrabinek gave us a crisp interview with much useful information. He himself had never been in hospital. He had managed to find only one ex-patient, Sergei Belov, who was willing to talk.

It's easy, given the long silence over Soviet psychiatry and the subterfuges I've just described, to be melodramatic. Belov's story is in many ways melodramatic. He isn't, however, representative of the majority of Soviet patients. Ludmilla, whose experiences I'll compare with Belov's, is much more typical. For her, Western policies aren't alluring but Western perfume is.

Belov – the dissident detective

Belov worked for the militia as both a detective and a lawyer. In the mid-seventies, he became involved in monitoring human rights activities, as he was allowed to do under the Helsinki Watch agreements. Belov insists that till then he had never seen a psychiatrist. He was as sane as anyone could be.

Belov never explained to me why he had suddenly become interested in human rights. As one of the militia, he knew it would be dangerous. Soon he became involved with underground publications. It didn't take long for the authorities to notice that the detective had turned dissident. Belov claims that he started to be harassed within months. He was taken to the *dispensaire*, or local health centre, for psychiatric assessment.

His behaviour allowed Soviet psychiatrists to use a convenient theory. Throughout the seventies, it was claimed that one symptom of schizophrenia was 'reformist delusions'. According to Dr Sidney Bloch, co-author of *Russia's Political Hospitals* (1977), to criticize the system was to invite being labelled as schizophrenic. Campaigning for change was proof of madness. Bloch points out that many dissidents had been accused of having 'reformist delusions' for making many of the criticisms Gorbachev is making now.

From 1978 onwards, the reform-minded Belov was frequently put in hospital for periods of four months. The detentions were limited for a reason Belov said. If you are hospitalized for more than four months, you become entitled to a pension. The state didn't want him to benefit and his activities weren't sufficiently serious to warrant a trial. However, he lost his job in the militia.

Then, in 1982, Belov was finally charged with anti-Soviet activities. Under article 190 of the Basic Law anyone who writes or publishes such material is guilty of a criminal offence. The court sent him to be assessed by a psychiatrist. It turned out to be a doctor who had seen him before during the period of harassment. The examination took a mere five minutes, Belov claims. The verdict was schizophrenia. Belov was sent to an ordinary psychiatric hospital and stayed there until 1983.

Then, one morning, Belov was told that he was moving. He was not told where. He was handcuffed after breakfast. He kept asking where he was going. Eventually, a sister said that he was going to a special hospital, a hospital for the criminally insane.

The USSR has sixteen special hospitals, at least. Bloch and Reddaway's *Russia's Political Hospitals* portrayed them as sinister institutions. Neither the brutality of the treatment nor the fact that there are inmates wrongly detained is remarkable. Both were certainly true of Britain's main special hospitals, Broadmoor and Rampton, in the seventies and early eighties. What is distinctive about the Soviet system is that a small proportion of the inmates have been convicted for activities that, in a democracy, are legal, normal and often mundane. Those sent there for anti-Soviet crimes were usually just expressing critical opinions about the political and economic system. Special hospitals house between 800 and 2,000 inmates each. About twelve to twenty inmates in each hospital were 'politicals'. For them, as sane people, to be sent to the madhouse was not merely unjust but a form of mental torture.

Belov's experiences in the special hospital at Volgograd were horrible. He shared a room with six to seven people. The discipline was strict. The food was poor and scarce. Relatives often found it hard to visit. Podrabinek said they were often frightened to ask about conditions because that might harm the chances of release. Fyodor Burlatsky, a senior journalist on the *Literary Gazette*, is now the chairman of the semi-official (and magnificently titled) Public Commission for Humanitarian Co-operation and Human Rights. Burlatsky understands relatives' problems. He told me that he had visited a friend of his in a special hospital near Moscow and had been utterly shocked by the condition he found him in.

For three-and-a-half years, Belov was in a punitive environment. He was never beaten up but he saw it happen to other inmates. Belov may have been perfectly sane when he went into hospital but he seemed marked by the experience. He was nervous and talked a great deal. It was hard to ask questions. He was immensely concerned that we should get his history in meticulous detail. None of these are signs of 'madness'. He didn't, when I talked to him for an hour, seem crazed, but a man who had been through gruelling experiences and was still recovering. It is very normal after a period of detention to need to talk about your experiences and to be furious about them. Belov seemed to me to be showing perfectly usual signs of that.

In October 1987, Belov left Volgograd Special Hospital for an ordinary hospital near Moscow. Then, in July 1988, he was finally released. He was one of the many political patients to benefit from the new atmosphere. Nevertheless, Belov is not entirely free. He is listed on a register of psychiatric patients. That is very restricting.

Belov said that when he was informed he was being put on the register, he didn't believe it. He asked if it meant he had to report to the authorities, 'To report as if I'm under surveillance.'

Belov claims that he was told, 'Yes, but you report to the

psychiatrist, not the police.' Every sixth day of the month he has to go to his local psychiatric health centre, called a *dispensaire*, and see his psychiatrist. It makes him feel very controlled, he said. He had protested against that as he had protested against being labelled as 'an invalid second class'. It was no consolation that because he was on the register, he got a small pension – fifty-five roubles a month.

The Soviet Union has never accepted that there was a policy of detaining politically awkward persons as patients. As a result, there have been no apologies and no compensation. Belov has asked for compensation because his flat was damaged by the militia. He also wanted to see the court record of his conviction. He couldn't obtain that. Initially, when he pointed out that over 500 roubles of damage had been done, he was told he might get compensation. But the local Soviet or City municipality decided he wasn't entitled. Belov laughed when he explained that the accountants told him that if they gave him any money, they'd lose it out of their salaries.

Belov chafes at the limits to his freedom. He has an invitation to see friends in West Germany but he has been denied permission to take it up.

Belov did get on the Helsinki Watch list but he was not a major dissident. There were no demonstrations or major campaigns in the West calling for his release. Rather, he is a typical, and convincing, example of the suffering caused by the abuse of psychiatry.

The majority of Soviet patients, however, have nothing to do with politics. In their focus on dissidents, Western journalists and psychiatrists ignored this silent majority.

There is no political mileage in dissecting their treatment and, once the dissident issue was firmly on the agenda in the early seventies, it seemed as if the only patients who mattered were political cases. Yet one can't understand how the political abuse occurred without understanding how Soviet psychiatry deals with other, apolitical patients. The mentally ill in any country rarely get the care or facilities they deserve partly because of ancient prejudices, and partly because there is little political pressure to better their lot. The Soviet Union is no exception.

Ludmilla, who can't lose her husband

Ludmilla is a good example of a totally apolitical patient. Her problems aren't to do with Marxism but with marriage. She is in her late forties and, as the photograph on her fussy dressing table shows, she was once beautiful. She is still concerned with her appearance. Pride of place on the dressing table is given to a bottle of Yardley Sea Spray, a scent that, like any Western cosmetic, is hard to get in the USSR. Ludmilla lives on the eighth floor of a block of flats outside Leningrad. It's a Russian tower block. The window at the entrance is broken; the lift is rickety. A slightly sour smell, cabbage and garbage mixed, hangs over the place. The tower block may be poor but it hasn't been defaced. In Britain and America, the walls of the corridor would be a riot of angry graffiti.

Ludmilla's flat consists of two rooms, a kitchen and a bathroom. She sleeps and lives in the big living room. She's done it rather nicely. As well as the dressing table, there's a cabinet full of pretty glasses. She has many books and pictures of her son who is in the army.

Ludmilla did not have a happy marriage and she is living with the consequences. Her husband treated her 'like a slave. I was always having to wash, cook and clean. He never responded to me as a woman.' It was hard in Russian to work out what she meant by this. Her husband had strange ideas. When Ludmilla became depressed, he kept nagging her not to take medicine. 'Only herbs help, he said,' she smiled condescendingly. 'He was very naïve.' Ludmilla now regards herself as something of an expert on medication.

Her husband has a drinking problem. In 1984, Ludmilla divorced him. She added that she had no regrets but was now 'afraid of loneliness because you're nothing without a man'. Her son, she said with pride, was a computer programmer with the army, a career soldier. She loved seeing him but it was hard for him to get away from Moscow so she did not see him too often. She repeatedly showed photographs of him. She shook her head sadly and she knew quite well he was never coming back to Leningrad.

The irony for Ludmilla is that her divorce has not freed her from her husband. In theory, when they got divorced, both partners were entitled to one-room flats of their own. There is, however, a chronic housing shortage. Four years after the divorce, Ludmilla's husband is still living in Ludmilla's flat. He now inhabits the second room. When we filmed, the door was firmly shut against us. It's clearly a miserable situation for her and she said that it contributed to her depression. There was no immediate prospect, however, of her getting a place that was really her own.

Ludmilla is on the register of psychiatric patients, like Belov. She spends her weekends at home and her week in the Bechterev Hospital. She likes the hospital as it's far from her husband and the routine there isn't very demanding. Moreover, she likes the feeling that she's being treated by quality doctors. Ludmilla doesn't approve of the doctors at her local health centre 'because I don't think they're well enough qualified'.

In Western psychiatry, which has become terribly cost-conscious, a person like Ludmilla would find it hard to qualify for a hospital bed. In the midst of Western debates on community care, it's clear that the ideal is a balanced system which has beds available when needed but doesn't teach patients to be helpless. The Soviet system has encouraged Ludmilla to become dependent on the hospital. It might be better to encourage her to resolve the situation with her husband. There is no question of Ludmilla being forced to have treatment she doesn't want but, with the collusion of the hospital, she is getting very used to being sick.

In this context, Ludmilla's attitude to being on the register of mental patients is interesting. She dislikes it but accepts it as inevitable if she is to get care.

Western journalists, campaigners and psychiatrists have had little interest in patients like her.

Abuse and ordinary treatment

Belov and Ludmilla have had very different experiences but there are still some important similarities between them. I want to argue that we can't understand what happened, and to some extent is still happening, to dissidents without understanding the whole structure of Soviet psychiatry. Bloch and Reddaway (1977) maintained there were two systems of Soviet psychiatry:

A system of abuse for political cases and decent care for the uncontroversial person. Bloch referred in an interview with me to the vast majority of 'innocent' Soviet psychiatrists. This division into many professional innocents and a few devilish leaders is too simple and too cosy an analysis. The political abuse would have been harder to arrange if there weren't some remarkably authoritarian features to the care of everyday patients – and few safeguards against that.

Western lawyers have been active in campaigning for patients' rights (Gostin 1977). In the Soviet Union, however, till recently, the law has been seen as a correct Socialist instrument in need of little reform. The state was benign in theory; its citizens didn't need protection from its wiles. Some lawyers fought tenaciously for dissident clients who had been charged with crimes but there wasn't a legal concept of suing the state for abuses or using such cases to alter the law. In any event, such a case could only have been brought through the Procurator General of the USSR, a high official of the Party and government. The current debate on how to improve Soviet laws so that citizens can employ them is very novel.

In every country, psychiatric patients suffer stigma and social disadvantage. The Soviet situation isn't exceptional but the USSR has been a society which prizes conformity. Such a society is likely to be particularly tough on the mentally ill. Throughout the book, I try to compare aspects of psychiatrists' behaviour to ordinary patients with their behaviour towards political ones. This presents parallels with the abuse of patients in non-socialist societies – a far from cosy topic that those who lambast Soviet psychiatry tend to skim past.

A rounded picture of present-day Soviet psychiatry is needed* because, after 1970, the West ignored important and

---

* Apart from Bloch and Reddaway's two books, there were two surveys by American psychiatrists in the 1960s (1960 and 1969). O'Connor published two useful surveys on Soviet psychology which included some material on psychiatry (O'Connor 1961 and 1966). Corson (1975) edited a good collection on USSR Psychology and Psychiatry. Lauterbach (1985) wrote a survey of Soviet psychotherapy. Valsiner in a thorough survey of developmental psychology (1988) touched on some psychiatric issues. There were far more books on Soviet psychology before 1970 when the dissident issue 'broke' (Cole and Maltzman 1968: Slobin 1966: Winn 1961). But there was little material on psychiatry and there hasn't been an attempt to give a rounded picture of Soviet psychiatry in the last twenty-five years.

positive aspects of Soviet psychiatry. There are things we can learn.

In the chapters that follow, I try to provide that picture, to see how Soviet psychiatry has changed under perestroika and glasnost and to examine the Soviet solutions to certain perennial problems such as how to make large psychiatric hospitals work well. In Chapter Two, I outline briefly the history of Soviet psychiatry and its current organization. In Chapter Three, I look at the Western accusations of political abuse, trying to bring the Bloch and Reddaway thesis up to date. In Chapter Four, I look at the system of *dispensaires* or health centres which offer the Soviet version of community care. In Chapter Five, I look at the work of ordinary hospitals, especially the work of the Kashenko Hospital in Moscow and the Kaluga Hospital. In Chapter Six, I look at the Serbsky Institute. It was here that many dissidents were diagnosed schizophrenic. In Chapter Seven, I examine the special hospital system. In Chapter Eight, I look at research institutes. In Chapter Nine, I examine the work of the new Commissions, set up under a new law, to which patients can appeal to get released. Finally, in Chapter Ten, I look at the politics of the World Psychiatric Association, ask whether, in the light of what we know, the Soviet Union should be readmitted and suggest ways in which international psychiatry could benefit from the controversy.

2

The Changing Structure of Psychiatry

Soviet psychiatry is changing essentially as a result of other, larger changes in Soviet society. Perestroika, the call for restructuring, and glasnost, the call for openness, have put quite new pressures on Soviet psychiatry. In this chapter, before dealing with the dissident issue, I want to sketch out some of these new legal, political and media pressures.

Throughout the seventies and eighties, Soviet psychiatrists acted as if they were outraged by allegations of the political misuse of psychiatry. It is telling to compare their reactions, then and now, to Western criticisms. In January 1983, a letter signed by Georgy Morosov and eighteen other psychiatrists explained why the Soviet Union had resigned from the World Psychiatric Association just before the Vienna Congress. It alleged that the State Department was engaged in a propaganda campaign to slander Soviet psychiatry. The letter spat sound and fury. There were no holds barred to its counter-allegations. It claimed that many Western psychiatrists had had the chance to examine 'patients in whom they were interested and no one expressed any doubts as to the correctness of the diagnosis'. In other words, Western doctors deceived their poor, innocent Soviet colleagues. Secondly, the letter claimed that Western psychiatrists 'hushed up' cases of émigrés who had complained of being unjustly detained and then, after leaving the Soviet Union, turned out to need psychiatric care. The perfidious West would stop at nothing. The letter accused the World Psychiatric Association of discrimination against the Soviet Union, of racism and of 'being an obedient tool in the hands of forces which are using psychiatry for their own political goals aimed at fanning up contradictions and enmity among psychiatrists of different countries'.

The letter made not the least concession to the allegations.

The withdrawal from the World Psychiatric Association didn't lead to any major known difficulties for the top Soviet psychiatrists. Dr Morosov remained as President of the Association of Neuropathologists and Psychiatrists, for example.

Soviet psychiatrists were excluded from some international conferences. Few were invited to speak at Western meetings. But they shrugged this off. Dr Vartanyan, a leading force in the negotiations, boasted to me, late in 1988, that they didn't miss the WPA. He was always jetting off to New York. He was running part of a major World Health Organization project into the biology of schizophrenia. The other main collaborating countries were Belgium and the USA.

Despite Vartanyan's bold front, the tone now is very different from that taken in 1983. Soviet psychiatrists regret the lack of co-operation. Painfully, a number of them explained that there had been 'misunderstandings'. It wasn't easy for West to understand East. They would be only too pleased to mend relations. That was one reason why my film was welcomed. Professor Nikolai Zharikov, the new president of the Soviet Association of Psychiatrists, insisted that, of course, they did not offer themselves for inspection to the West. No reputable body of psychiatrists could brook such interference in their internal affairs. But they were minded to be conciliatory. This mood isn't, however, the result of a change of heart by the profession. Soviet psychiatry has been unable to isolate itself from political upheavals. By 1986, psychiatry remained one of the leading sores in the Soviet human rights record. Every political dissident held in a psychiatric hospital, every prisoner of conscience made it harder for Gorbachev to persuade the West that the Soviet Union was really changing. The psychiatric detention of dissidents had become counter-productive.

The access I was given was part of a deliberate programme to get the best propaganda value out of real reform. However, it has not been easy to launch such reforms and will not be easy to consolidate them. Many psychiatrists find them threatening, not because they were 'guilty' of misdiagnosing dissidents but because the reforms require a rather new approach to all patients.

Here I offer some background to the new climate;

A brief account of some historical developments.

'There was in old Russia', said Burlatsky, 'a fine tradition of humane psychiatry.' St Basil, whose cathedral dominates Red Square, believed the mentally ill deserved special care. To be touched in the mind was to be touched by God. In *The Idiot*, Dostoevsky created a holy fool, saint, innocent and lunatic. Such traditions, I was told, showed how wrong it was to pillory the Russians, old and new alike, for cruelty to the mentally ill.

Psychiatry developed later in the Soviet Union than it did in Britain or America. By the 1850s, for example, Britain, America and France had well-established mental hospitals. A good account of them is to be found in Digby (1986) or Porter (1989). As people moved into towns during the Industrial Revolution, it was less and less possible to keep the village idiot in the village. The demands of town life required some secure institution where they didn't trouble folk going about their now busy lives. The Soviet Union remained a rural country well into the 1900s. A few monasteries that provided asylum. Peter the Great decreed in 1723 that asylums should be built. The first small asylum, with 25 beds, was opened in 1776 under Catherine the Great. In 1809, the first true Russian psychiatric hospital was founded. As late as 1910, there were few mental hospitals and only 438 psychiatrists in all the Tsar's kingdoms (O'Connor 1966).

The main Moscow psychiatric hospital, the Kashenko, wasn't completed till 1894 when a million gold roubles were collected by public subscription. The main Leningrad mental hospital, the Bechterev, wasn't established till 1908. Two of the other oldest institutions in the USSR were founded around that time – the Rimsky Korsakov Institute in 1889 and the Serbsky Institute of General and Forensic Psychiatry in 1921.

Psychiatry also had a very particular scientific slant. In nearly all psychiatric hospitals today, portraits of Pavlov stare down from the walls. Pavlov (1849–1936) first became known in the West for his experiments on conditioning. His research showing how dogs could be made to salivate to a bell because they associated it with food influenced American psychology enormously. Pavlov seemed to have revealed the components of behaviour. He affected the development of learning theory (Hill 1988). Many behaviourists came to argue that mental illness was the result of inappropriate learning. Pavlov, however, took a more biological line. He stressed the importance of organic factors in psychiatric illness. His ideas came to dominate Soviet psychiatry after the Revolution. In many ways, that was peculiar.

According to Marxist-Leninism, human beings are social animals, products of class and social relationships. Personality is the result of interaction between the individual and social forces. If I am depressed, it can't really be my fault because my depression must be caused partly, at least, by society. After the Revolution, many wild, abandoned young people roamed a chaotic Russia. Eventually, they were 'retrained' to play their part in society. According to Valsiner (1988) no one felt these young people were responsible for their delinquency. Social forces were blamed in a coherent Marxist fashion.

With such a political theory, it is remarkable that Pavlov's biological ideas not only survived but became so dominant. Partly it was due to Pavlov's prestige. He won the Nobel Prize in 1904: his work was internationally famous largely because it had been used in America by John B. Watson to promote behaviourism. Pavlov and his supporters were also adept academic politicians. They controlled election to the USSR Academy of Medicine and the USSR Academy of Sciences. In 1950, fourteen years after Pavlov died, a famous joint meeting of the two Academies castigated psychiatry for deviations from Pavlov's ideas. Theoretical opponents were nervous. Meyassechev, the Director of the Bechterev Institute in Leningrad, who supported the development of psychotherapy, did not dare offer himself for election. The Pavlov faction hated his anti-biological position and would block his election. Instead Meyassechev had himself elected to the Academy of Education. In 1966, the climate was more liberal and he could finally complain of how unfair it was that someone with his views had been accused of 'anti-Pavlov fabrications'. These were not ivory tower battles. The great child psychologist Vygotsky ended up out of favour, out of Moscow and, nearly, out of work.

From the early fifties, Soviet psychiatry came to be dominated by A. Z. Snezhnevsky. He became director of the Moscow Institute of Psychiatry, a post which interestingly has not been filled since his death in 1986. One Novosti represent-ative quipped to Julian Goodburn that Snezhnevsky was 'the hangman'. Snezhnevsky developed the concept of sluggish schizophrenia (a form of schizophrenia where the symptoms are subtle, latent or only apparent to the skilled eye of the psychiatrist) and he was certainly seen in the West as an arch villain. He never challenged the emphasis on the biological and organic. Academic controversies – is it nature or nurture that determines behaviour? – have a human impact in psychiatry. Theories that blame social conditions for mental illness see the patient as a victim. He or she deserves care and tenderness. The fault lies outside the person. But if the fault is organic, then it lies within the person. They are perceived as, somehow, more responsible and more to blame for their condition. They deserve less. This isn't logic but psycho-logic. Common sense tells me I am no more to blame for the bad genes that 'cause' schizophrenia than for the genes that give me blue eyes. But common sense doesn't prevail easily when discussing mental illness. It is no accident that much of the language still used to describe it arose in the nineteenth century and is pejorative. Someone is *de-ranged* or out of their mind or *alienated*.

The tone taken towards patients in much Soviet writing highlights their deficiencies. For example, in *The Pictorial Language of Schizophrenics* (1982), Morosov and his co-authors accuse 'sick artists' of being only interested in the baser parts of life. Their drawings betray 'deformation and distortion' which is 'intimately related to the basic manifestations of the disease'. These patients are so incompetent that they 'cannot even complete secondary education, learn a trade, hold a job; oddities of dressing, untidiness and sloppiness appear'. The contempt expressed is remarkable; so is the lack of compassion.

This theoretical slant, seeing the patient as bad and to blame, affects treatment. Patients are rarely seen as individuals but as 'medical objects' who should be grateful to have expertise lavished on them. Doctors are not used to dealing with them as equal human beings who have every right to have a say in their treatment. In much psychiatry, the medical model of psychiatric illness has been questioned, but there is no sign of that either in current Soviet practice or theory. Paramedical professions are weak: social work is not recognized as a profession; psychologists are meek; nurses deferential. Few dare question medical authority. Pavlov rules – yet.

The Revolution, however, did change the provision of health care. Before 1917, doctors were for the rich. The Revolution committed itself to provide medical care for everyone, a guarantee enshrined in the first Soviet Constitution and in all later revisions.

In 1921, a system of local health centres called *dispensaires* was set up which came to specialize in psychiatry. The first ones were in Moscow and Leningrad. By 1957, there were 2,300 psychiatric *dispensaires* inside general health centres and 119 special psychiatric ones. Since then, there has been rapid development of the psychiatric *dispensaires*. They became local mental health centres, much like those set up under Kennedy's initiative in 1963.

Every small town has a *dispensaire* and in big cities each borough has one. In outlying areas like in Siberia, one *dispensaire* will cover a vast catchment area. The system provides free and accessible health care. The decision to promote *dispensaires* wasn't just idealistic, though.

The Soviet Constitution provides a key to the understanding of Soviet psychiatry. In the West, our tradition of human rights pits the citizen against the State. Very occasionally, a politician will, like John Kennedy, ask us to think what we can do for our country. But, in general, we have rights without any major duties other than the duty to obey the law. If I wish to live as a tramp or to devote my life to a study of butterflies, it's my business and my right to do so as long as I hurt no one else. The Soviet constitution proclaims a rather different relationship. The citizen is meant to be a productive member of the socialist community. If I choose to be a tramp or butterfly-maniac, I am hurting others because I am depriving the State of my labour. This is not necessarily bad, just odd given Western traditions. But being a 'parasite' is an actual crime much like being a vagrant was in Tudor England.

This emphasis meant doctors had to get citizens fit and see the idle were not malingering. The doctor became an agent of social control. The ethical concerns of Western medicine such as the right to confidential treatment didn't have quite the same priority. The *dispensaire* system offered a basis for checking not just on the sick but on those who were lazy or didn't conform. It was to make for an exceptionally interfering sort of medicine.

The register system

Early on, the *dispensaires* began to keep a register of psychiatric patients. According to some authorities there are two registers – one of ordinary patients and the second of the specially aggressive. Nearly all the patients whose case histories form part of this book are on the register. In theory, psychiatrists can place a patient on it if she or he is a danger either to themselves or to society. What is most striking is the sheer number of people who are on the register and who, at some point, have been deemed 'socially dangerous'. At the end of 1987, some 5.5 million people were on it and 1.8 million of them were diagnosed as schizophrenics. The rest were border-line cases or had personality problems and about 1.7 million were described as 'feeble-minded'. This did not include the mentally handicapped, but those who were 'socially inadequate'.

The figures are, frankly, staggering. In Britain, 17,000 people a year are compulsorily put into hospital, usually for short periods of time. In Japan, in many ways the country with the worst human rights record in psychiatry, 330,000 are in hospi-tal, 80 per cent held against their will. It's true that not all the 5.5 million on the Soviet register are in hospital but they are all liable to be sent there. And, once someone is on the register, it is not easy to get taken off. Most *dispensaires* insist a person must spend five years free of any sign of psychiatric illness before they are removed.

In a time of change, as now, it is hard to pin down just what restrictions being on the register imposes. Some are formal, others are informal. Anyone on the register has to be super-vised by their *dispensaire*. They are on perpetual probation. Just how actively a particular patient is supervised depends on many things, including the severity of his symptoms, what his family say, what his neighbours say and the judgement of doctors. I was told that the information that someone was on the register was kept confidential. But many patients complained everyone in their community knew they were on it. The *dispensaires* often telephone family, friends or places of work to check how someone is doing. This helps create stigma. Many of the patients I talked to said they felt ashamed of their status. It dented their self-esteem and self-confidence.

The biological model sees the patient as defective; the health system labels him as a social danger. The register also leads to more tangible losses. In the first Soviet Constitution, mental patients lost their right to vote in elections. So did convicts, monks and relatives of the Tsar. The insane are the only group who still haven't got the vote back. The 1977 Constitution offered them nothing. In Britain, patients now have the vote. The restrictions patients told me still applied to them as a result of being on the register included: not being able to travel abroad; not being allowed to hold certain jobs; having to report regularly to the *dispensaire*; having to accept the treatment and drugs the *dispensaire* decided on; and being liable to be recalled to hospital at any time.

One patient, Irina, said, 'people at work treat you as an idiot if they know you are on the register. I lost my relationship too as a result of that.' Ludmilla said that she was 'on the list, unfortunately'. Irina wanted to be taken off the list but she believed that if she were, she couldn't get treatment if she needed it.

In every country, the mentally ill face prejudice. In the Soviet Union, the register feeds that prejudice. Dr Egorov, the Director General of Psychiatry and Neurology at the Ministry of Health, accepted that the list had been defined in a very wide way.

He said: 'The main trend involved a strict system of putting the mentally ill on the register, a strict system of monitoring their behaviour and the adoption of maximum possible measures to exclude socially dangerous acts.' Staff in psychiatric hospitals and clinics were given an extra 30 per cent on their salaries compared to other medical personnel essentially as danger money. One of the nagging concerns mentioned by some psychiatrists was whether they would now lose this bonus.

Dr Egorov conceded that, 'It must be said that the term

"socially dangerous" was understood in a very broad sense and included a very broad spectrum.' He went so far as to give an example which fringed on political abuse. Dr Egorov said:

Coming back to the issue of possible abuses, I remembered that a few days ago our magazine *Arguments and Facts* reported that the so-called preventive hospitalization of mentally ill persons on the eve of some major national celebrations or political events had been wide-spread. In other words, before those major events or celebrations were to take place, groups of socially dangerous, ill persons who were on the list at every mental hospital, used to be taken to psychiatric hospitals just in case, as the saying goes, so that they would not commit anything improper, God forbid. But I would not, perhaps, call it malice or abuse. Therefore, we are aware that there is great interest abroad in the processes currently underway in our country, and, as far as I know, there is a lot of goodwill. Therefore, we think that our foreign colleagues – psychiatrists, including British psychiatrists – will have equal understanding and benevolence for the changes now taking place in our psychiatry, the more so as we have no secrets and are prepared to show everything that would clarify the present-day situation.

This wide definition of the mentally ill had little to do with suppressing dissent, Dr Egorov argued. Rather, it reflected the caution and conservatism of doctors. Dr Marat Vartanyan claimed that Soviet psychiatry worked very much to a 'medical model, not a juridical model' as in the West. The juridical model emphasized the rights of patients: the medical model emphasized their need for treatment and saw doctors as competent to impose treatment. Psychiatric patients were not the best judges of what they needed.

Ordinary patients have been far more affected than political ones by the register, though it has been used to keep a check on political cases. In some cases, that practice still continues. In general, Dr Egorov accepted that the register had helped make the public fear both the mentally ill and psychiatry.

As part of the new liberal climate, the Ministry of Health is hoping to diminish the numbers on the register. In five large areas, including Leningrad and Moscow, the aim is to reduce the numbers on the register by 20 per cent. Dr Egorov said it was too early to say how that experiment was going but he had high hopes.

Hopes are nice but imprecise. Yet, one needs plenty of precision in assessing changes. At Kaluga Mental Hospital I was told that, even during the bad Brezhnev years, they had taken many people off the register. Dr Lifschitz, Kaluga's director, had hit on the happy innovation of moving the *dispensaire* into the hospital. One doctor would care for the patient both in the community and in hospital. Lifschitz argued that this had helped reduce the numbers on the register since 1972. I asked for an exact breakdown and, very courteously, Dr Lifschitz provided it. The breakdown told a slightly different story. Certainly, every year, between 200 and 500 left the register. But also each year, large numbers of new patients were put on it. The balance sheet which Dr Lifschitz presented showed that in 1972 there had been just over 2,500 patients on the Kaluga register and in 1988 there were 2,405. He had accelerated the turnover but not really reduced the numbers. I do not mean to accuse Dr Lifschitz of dishonesty. It was very open of him to reveal the details of his data but that data did not quite prove what he, and others, said it did. Many experts in the Soviet Union thought Kaluga had the magic formula for reducing the register. Progress in the five areas Dr Egorov mentioned needs to be carefully monitored.

Despite the new emphasis on reform, no Soviet psychiatrist I talked to questioned the need for a register of millions.

The media

The failure to report psychiatry was the result both of censorship and conservatism. Dr Kosirev of the Kashenko Hospital told me that in 1969 he had helped a journalist gather material for an in-depth study of psychiatry for the *Literary Gazette*. Kosirev had been very disappointed when it had been banned by the censor. Eleonora Gorbunova, Novosti's health correspondent, told me that when she visited the UK she was amazed to see a programme on TV about still-births. No one could possibly make such a programme in the Soviet Union. It would be too shocking.

The effect of Western accusations on Soviet psychiatry was to make it virtually impossible for Soviet journalists to write about any aspect of psychiatry. Marat Vartanyan said, 'There was a taboo on psychiatry. It was not an issue that could be discussed for the last fifteen or twenty years.' Anatoly Potapov, the Minister of Health of the Russian Republic, a burly man who looks eerily like Khrushchev, has stated that psychiatry 'has for a long time remained not only without a thorough assessment of its shortcomings but also without adequate coverage of its problems in the mass circulation press'. Potapov said that one problem was that of confidentiality, but he added that, 'The state of affairs in psychiatry . . . needs not only attention but constant monitoring on the part of the public.' Potapov added that the press and public could do much 'to remove the shortcomings built up over many years, improving the material base, altering the work style and developing progressive new forms of help'. Potapov stressed that no new psychiatric hospital had been built in five years even though hospitals were badly overcrowded. The organization of care was poor. He added, 'The composition of leading cadres is causing concern and there are large numbers of cases of breaches of labour discipline and drunkenness.' (Interview in *Digest of the Soviet Press*).

When I met Dr Potapov, he lambasted the quality of psychiatrists and other doctors. Many were incompetent and should, he growled, be dismissed. I found it remarkable that he should vouchsafe these outspoken views to a foreign journalist.

Soviet journalists confirmed there had been a taboo yet insisted that it had not been imposed by any decree or institution. You just knew that this wasn't the kind of subject you tackled. Andrei Mann of the *Medical Gazette*, who I had arranged to interview independently, said, 'Psychiatry was seen as a dangerous subject. To write the kind of articles that I wrote about corruption and bribe-taking at the Kashenko or the kind of articles that Andrianov wrote in *Socialist Industry* wouldn't have been possible before.'

The situation began to change in 1986 with Mann and Andrianov both writing articles on corruption at the Kashenko Hospital in Moscow. There, doctors were willing to diagnose sane criminals as mad so that they could avoid going to prison. After a year, quietly, the patients would be found cured and released. In 1987, *Komsomolskaya Pravda* alleged even more fundamental abuse claiming that a patient had been unjustly hospitalized. This article led to a furore. The information in it was largely untrue. Much of the evidence came from a psychiatrist who was found to be himself disturbed. Mann investigated the story and said that it was just a series of mistakes – an estimate I tend to believe.

The publication of the *Komsomolskaya Pravda* piece was significant though, in the end, the discrediting of the exposé suited conservative doctors. Vartanyan said it showed how irresponsible the Soviet press was. Professor Modest Kabanov, director of the Bechterev Institute, said it showed how poorly equipped Soviet journalists were to deal with such issues. 'It was not professional,' he said. Even Dr Chasov, the USSR Minister of Health, complained bitterly of that article. In an interview on Soviet Television on the programme *Health* (22 November 1987) he said he didn't understand why the journalists hadn't sought official comments on the complaints they reported. 'When you read the article, you think surely the correspondent could have at least come to see the deputy minister to find out that back on 2 April there was an expanded collegium of the USSR Ministry of Health at which all the issues raised were examined.' If the journalists had only done that, then 'everything would be clear and understandable'. Those who criticize the Soviet media don't admit they could hardly expect a repressive system to produce instant perfect investigative journalism when, miraculously, it was suddenly allowed. Some psychiatrists carped that Soviet journalists were as inaccurate as Western ones. Dr Vartanyan and Dr Zharikov, the new President of the Soviet Association of Psychiatrists, were both now convinced the media did have a role to play, educating the public that had been so deprived of information. Instead of rising to this noble task, muckraking journalists were gunning for psychiatry. In the process, they were inciting not just ridicule but hatred. Psychiatrists had become victims. One of Vartanyan's smart quips is that psychiatric abuse now means abuse of psychiatrists. 'There are graffiti', he commented with a sigh, 'which say "kill psychiatrists" and naturally that upsets us very much.' He added that they earned their 30 per cent bonus more than ever now. In the good old days, posters would have celebrated the socialist shrink triumphant.

Senior psychiatrists may not like what the media writes, but it does not follow that the media can tackle any topic. Even now, there are limits. So far, no article has tackled, from the Soviet perspective, the allegations about abuse of dissidents. That area remains taboo. Andrei Mann told me that he had made some preliminary inquiries during a trip to Leningrad. He was careful how he put it. 'It would be wrong to say I met hindrance,' he said, 'but the reaction of psychiatrists, academicians and scientists was over-sensitive.' They were touchy because psychiatry was a dark subject and also because with re-entry to the WPA in the air, they felt everyone had to rally round. 'Articles of the sort I was talking about would not be helpful, I was told.' So far, Mann has not published anything on that theme.

Just as the media is not totally free, so the new laws are not totally perfect as far as patients' rights are concerned.

Legal rights

Today, Soviet psychiatrists are bitter about press coverage and ambivalent about the new law of January 1988. Many said both that the law was a sign of progress and that it made them nervous. Yet this new law is hardly a liberal dream. Both in theory and in practice, it has many limitations. The safeguards it offers patients are somewhat incomplete.

Organizationally, the new law requires local health authorities to create the post of Chief Psychiatrist. The Chief Psychiatrist is supposed to supervise and administer psychiatry in his area. He has competing duties. First to 'take measures to protect the rights and lawful interests of persons suffering from mental disorder' and second 'to protect society from dangerous actions by the mentally ill'. He has to balance the rival interests of the individual and society. One of his functions under the 1988 law is to hear the appeals of patients and their families.

The new law has many positive aspects. It guarantees patients free medical care and 'a respectful and humane approach without any infringement of the patient's human dignity'.

Patients are entitled to social and legal assistance and 'the help of a lawyer to safeguard their rights and interests'. The patient may ask for any psychiatrist employed by the local health authority to take part in the Commission that will decide whether or not they are to stay on the register or in hospital.

The new law is strict about the duties of doctors. The psychiatrist must act independently and must be guided 'solely by medical criteria and the law'. The doctor must introduce himself to the person he is examining quite formally to leave no doubt concerning what is at stake in the psychiatric examination. The confidentiality of information given by the patient must be respected.

But Section 9 of the new law is not quite as respectful of patients' rights. It reads, 'A person whose actions give sufficient grounds to conclude that he is suffering from a mental disorder and which disrupt social order or infringe the rules of the socialist community and also constitute a direct danger to himself and those around him may be subject to an initial psychiatric examination without his consent.' The key ambiguous phrase is 'the rules of the socialist community'. It was just because they infringed the rules of the socialist community that dissidents found themselves in trouble. This phrase about 'socialist rules' clearly leaves the way open for all kinds of pressure to be brought on patients.

In most democratic countries, at least two professionals have to agree in order to commit a patient. Western legal systems (after many campaigns) now usually insist that the patient is given reasons for being detained. In Japan, there was much criticism of the fact that before 1987 someone could be committed just on the evidence of one psychiatrist. The new Soviet law, however, also allows one lone psychiatrist to commit. It reads as if that is to be the normal practice. Only after a person has been committed are other experts invited to get involved.

After taking someone to hospital, the psychiatrist must inform the family and the area's Chief Psychiatrist. Rather oddly, section 16 says that the psychiatrist *must* (my italics) get the assistance of 'organs of internal affairs' in effecting the hospitalization. These 'organs' seem to refer to the Ministry of the Interior which runs the police force. In other words, when anyone is taken to hospital, the police must know. Within twenty-four hours, the patient must be examined by a commission of psychiatrists. The law doesn't define how many psychiatrists make a commission, but, in practice, I was told it was two or three. If the commission decides not to discharge the patient, it has to send their papers to the office of the Chief Psychiatrist. He has to ratify the decision usually without seeing the patient. Patients can appeal to the Chief Psychiatrist. If he was the psychiatrist who signed the committal order, then the patient can appeal to the Chief Psychiatrist of the next larger authority.

The patient has to be examined by a commission every month to see if it is necessary to continue compulsory treatment. Even patients who come voluntarily into hospital (which is rare) may lose that status and be detained. Section 20 stresses that if their mental state is judged to constitute a 'direct danger to themselves or those around them' they will be denied discharge.

The penalties for failing to carry out these provisions are severe, apparently, for 'the internment in a psychiatric hospital of a person known to be mentally healthy is a criminal offence in accordance with the law of the Union Republics'. The particular law that this offends is the law against the unjust imprisonment by officials and, in theory, it could have been used before 1988. Fyodor Burlatsky said that he knew of no case where a doctor had ever been charged with this offence.

What is striking about the new law – and we shall see how it works in practice in Chapter Nine – is that all these decisions are taken by psychiatrists. No other disciplines are involved. In Britain, for example, from 1959 onwards a patient could only be committed if a doctor and a social worker agreed that he or she was likely to be a danger to themselves or others. Two different disciplines would provide some degree of protection. Patients in Britain could also involve lawyers from the moment they were threatened with committal. The Mental Health Law Commission which supervises the detention of patients in Britain was first headed by a peer, Lord Colville and is now headed by a lawyer, Louis Blom Cooper. For all its liberality, the new Soviet law still leaves power very much in the hands of psychiatrists. It is only at the very end of the process that a patient can involve the courts and lawyers. This right is given in Sections 27 and 28.

They say that: 'The actions of a Chief Psychiatrist may be appealed against by the person with respect to whom they were committed as well as by his representatives in accordance with the USSR law on Procedures for Appealing to the Courts Unlawful Actions by Officials that Infringe the Rights of Citizens.' The appeal may be either to the Chief Psychiatrist of the higher-level public health agency and then to a court or directly to the court. 'The Procurator General of the Soviet Union has the obligation to see that such committals are carried out legally.' (*Current Digest of the Soviet Press*, no. 6, 1988, p. 13).

This right to appeal to the court is being presented as radically novel. In an interview with *Isvestia* (15 January 1988) Ivan Samoshchenko, USSR First Deputy Minister of Justice, said, 'In general this opportunity to appeal against the actions of psychiatrists is something new for our legislation. It will serve as a serious obstacle to abuse.' Technically, however, the right to appeal to courts existed as part of the Basic Law of the USSR that was formulated under Stalin. In fact, in many of the most famous dissident cases like that of Medvedev, groups of citizens asked the Procurator General to intervene. In some cases, the tactic worked.

It is too early to say how well the new law will work. In Chapter Eight, I analyse a number of current cases. But even in its structure, the law isn't quite the liberal measure it is being presented as.

There are other indications of progress with legal reforms, however. For some years, the United Nations Commission on Human Rights has had a subcommittee working on a draft document aimed at protecting the mentally ill. One obstacle to progress has been the attitude of the Soviet Union. In August 1988, however, the Soviet Union finally accepted and signed a document which provides an excellent basis for protecting patients' rights. The 1988 document (UN Economic and Social Council: Human Rights and Scientific and Technological

Developments) insists that patients will be treated 'with human-
ity and respect'. They will not be discriminated against. They
will have the right to appoint legal representatives. A patient
will only be detained if he will cause harm to himself and 'it is
in the person's best interests to be admitted' or 'will cause
serious harm to other people'. Detention is also allowed if an
individual is in too bad a condition to consent to a treatment
which can only be given in a hospital.

There are some provisions which are phrased in such a way
as to make one suppose that they are aimed especially at the
kinds of abuse that happened in the USSR. Article 6 states in
Section 1: 'A diagnosis that a person has a mental illness shall
be in accordance with internationally accepted medical standards.' Many Soviet dissidents were said to suffer from 'sluggish
schizophrenia', a variety of disease not recognized in most
other countries. Section 3 of Article 6 states that, 'No person
shall be labelled, diagnosed or treated as mentally ill for
political, economic, social, cultural, racial or religious reasons
or for reasons of family conflict or for any other reasons not
directly relevant to his mental health status.' The implications
of this are spelled out in Section 4. 'Non-conformity with
moral, social, cultural or political values or religious beliefs
prevailing in a person's community shall never be a determining
factor in diagnosing mental illness.' The Soviet Union's signing
of the Working Party document has been hailed as yet another
sign of a new mood in psychiatry.

Again, a critical perspective is important. Marat Vartanyan
said that he thought psychiatrists the world over would find this
UN paper an impossible document and would campaign against
it. As things are, in some details, the Soviet law passed in
January 1988 does not meet its criteria. One important provision of the UN document (Article 22) is that countries should
set up 'an independent multi-disciplinary commission with
responsibility for promoting compliance with the Principles and
Guarantees as enacted in national law: to inspect and monitor
the procedures used in dealing with patients and the conditions
in which they are treated and to investigate and make recom-
mendations concerning complaints by patients and their representatives'. There's no sign of the setting up in the Soviet Union

of such a multi-disciplinary body which would boost the standing of the non-medical professions.

Few Soviet psychiatrists apart from Vartanyan seem to have made themselves familiar with this UN document. Few were delighted with the new law, even though it did not even mention multi-disciplinary commissions. In sum, there was no sign of psychiatrists being willing to share their power.

It would be churlish to deny the progress that has been made. There is considerable political desire to reform psychiatry in the Soviet Union. The media can now write about most aspects of psychiatry. The new law provides some protections. But the reforms so far are rather limited. In the next chapter we shall see that the position with regard to political patients has improved but that many difficulties remain. Furthermore, at the risk of sounding cynical, it has to be remembered that all these reforms are being flaunted at a time when the Soviet Union wants to become a respectable member of international psychiatry. I don't suggest they are mere window dressing but it is no accident that they are being carried out now. However, the reforms won't work unless Soviet psychiatrists change many of their attitudes and practices. That will not be easy as the ambiguous reactions of Soviet psychiatrists to the recent semi-liberal measures show.

3
The Dissident Debate

The treatment meted out to dissidents is best illustrated by a real case. Major General Grigorenko came to be one of the most famous dissidents.

Grigorenko had had a distinguished military career. In 1965, he became interested in the cause of the Crimean Tartars. The Tartars had been persecuted under Stalin. They were campaigning for the preservation of their culture and some control of their lands. Grigorenko's activities began to worry the KGB and in May 1969 he was set up. He was telephoned and asked to come to Tashkent to be a character witness in the trial of some Tartar nationalists. He went and was himself arrested at Tashkent airport. It would have been embarrassing to charge a Major General with anti-Soviet activities so the KGB resorted to the use of psychiatry. The first examination took place in August 1969 on KGB premises in Tashkent. To the KGB's dismay, the commission, under Professor Detengof, found Grigorenko was responsible for his actions and argued that there was no need to admit him as a patient to deepen the diagnosis. The KGB then flew Grigorenko to Moscow and had him examined at the Serbsky. The commission headed by Dr G. Morosov, V. M. Morosov and D. R. Lunts concluded more helpfully that Grigorenko was 'suffering from a mental illness in the form of a pathological paranoid development of the personality with the presence of reformist ideas that have appeared in his personality' (quoted by Bloch and Reddaway, 1977, p. 112). The Serbsky commission smoothed the way to a quick and quiet solution. Grigorenko was certified insane. He could not appear at his trial in Tashkent since he had been declared 'too ill' to defend himself. Grigorenko was found not responsible for his criminal acts, disseminating deliberate fabrications which defamed the USSR. He was sent to Chernyakhovsk Special Hospital where he spent nearly four years. His case and those of Bukovsky and Medvedev (which I examine below) put psychiatric abuse in the USSR firmly on the international human rights agenda. The notes on Grigorenko's psychiatric examination were first published in the West in 1970.

Until the late sixties, no one publicized old examples of political abuse. Nicholas I had carted off one rebel to a Moscow asylum as early as 1835. The ex-President of Estonia, Pacts, was detained from 1941 to 1956 in Kazan Special Hospital as were other cases. But there was little controversy. Reports by American psychiatrists in 1960 and 1969 on Soviet psychiatry in general were basically positive, praising the community care system. In 1966, the International Congress of Psychologists met in Moscow. Sessions were addressed by many forensic psychiatrists including Dr Lunts and Dr Gregory Morosov. Dan Slobin, professor of psychology at Iowa, who edited a guide to the Congress, quoted them as perfectly reputable sources. The first mention of the issue came in Tarsis' novel *Ward 7* (published in the West in 1965). It built on Chekhov's story *Ward 6* but its criticisms were part of a fiction, not documented fact.

In 1970, a number of worried letters appeared in the *American Journal of Psychiatry* and a harsh, but short, article on 'Soviet Mental Prisons' was published by S. P. Pisarev (Survey no 77 pp. 175–80). Segal (1976) in a useful article argues that the Soviet regime felt it could no longer put dissidents in Stalinist concentration camps. That looked too bad in the West. As a result, Segal suggests, the KGB began to involve psychiatrists in some cases. The question of the political abuse of psychiatry finally 'took off' between 1970 and 1972.

In 1970, two very different kinds of evidence appeared. First there was the testimony of the biologist, Zhores Medvedev. In his book, written with his brother Roy (1971), Zhores Medvedev told the story of how he had been committed to the Kaluga Mental Hospital after he had started to question why it was so hard to get journals from the West and asked to be allowed to travel there. Medvedev described how he had been

committed to the hospital after he had refused to submit to a
voluntary psychiatric examination. He noted that Dr Lifschitz
'tried his best to sound friendly and convincing but sometimes
there was a threatening note:' After a while, a police major
entered Medvedev's house and demanded 'What's this? Why
are you refusing to submit to the requests of the doctor?'
Medvedev asked who this major was and pointed out that he
had no authority to demand anything. Police Major Nemov
then retorted 'We are responsible for enforcement' and, thump-
ing his chest, shouted 'Get to your feet. I order you to get to
your feet.' (p. 36) Medvedev was taken to Kaluga. His incarceration did not last long. After nineteen days, and a welter of
internal and external protest – he was released. There was
massive daily coverage in the international press.

The other case to receive great publicity was that of Vladimir
Bukovsky. In July 1970 he was interviewed in Moscow by
William Cole, a CBS television correspondent. Bukovsky
talked of how he had been harassed, arrested and diagnosed
mentally ill repeatedly because of his human rights work.
Bukovsky had long periods in the Serbsky and in Leningrad
Special Hospital. In January 1971, Bukovsky appealed to
Western psychiatrists with evidence of cases of unjust detention. He wanted world psychiatry to censure the USSR. Psychiatrists are always hesitant to criticize each other and Bukovsky's
plea to the Congress of the World Psychiatric Association in
Mexico didn't even result in a proper discussion. Bloch and
Reddaway denounced the procedural games that made this
possible: 'Other psychiatrists expressed concern but saw it as a
political problem and therefore not an appropriate matter for a
scientific meeting within the purview of the WPA.' The WPA
officials were annoyed that pamphlets outlining the dissidents'
case had been distributed. Such a contempt for scientific
matters, bringing impure politics into it was denounced as 'an
attempt to involve a scientific association in the cold war'.
(Quoted by Bloch and Reddaway 1977 p. 92).

The Congress's unwillingness to even consider the evidence
did not impress the liberal press. Two journalists in particular,
I. F. Stone and Bernard Levin, thundered at the complacency
of international psychiatry.

The Soviet Union made some attempt to defend itself against

what they called unjust accusations but the West continued to publicize many cases like Grigorenko.

Individual cases aroused much sympathy and protest. Bukovsky was probably the first to suggest that there was a systematic policy of using psychiatry against dissent. Bukovsky, who had suffered mightily, argued, not surprisingly, that Soviet psychiatrists knew quite well what they were doing. They were acting for the regime, deliberately perverting the medical ethic. Bukovsky's view was attractive to many in the West. A slightly different view was articulated by Boris Segal, a psychiatrist who emigrated from Moscow to Boston. Segal argued that if there was such a policy it was muddled. The KGB would refer dissidents to psychiatrists. Segal wrote (1976): 'Often when the KGB or other party organs questioned psychiatrists about the existence of mental disorder in a particular dissenter they frequently received positive responses based on undefined criteria of mental illness. In many cases, one cannot clearly see a conscious evil design of the KGB or psychiatrists. Very few psychiatrists "discover" mental illness only to serve the authorities and to punish the liberals.' (p. 273).

Segal suggested that the KGB didn't order doctors to diagnose dissidents as mad. The psychiatrists were conformist rather than cowed. They had no sympathy with dissidence. As bureaucrats they knew that normal persons didn't get involved in political controversy. If you did, you were looking for trouble. That in itself suggested a certain abnormality. Segal did not seek to condone Soviet psychiatrists but he tried to explain their behaviour without demonizing it. He also linked their treatment of dissidents with their treatment of other patients. A bureaucratic arrogance permeated both.

Segal was writing in an obscure academic book, however. His interesting interpretation was largely forgotten when a major study appeared in 1977. It focused most of the available information to devastating effect.

Sidney Bloch, a psychiatrist, and Peter Reddaway, a political expert on the Soviet Union, published *Russia's Political Hospitals* (1977). In that, and in *Soviet Psychiatric Abuse* (1984), they argued a formidable case. They claimed there was a systematic use of psychiatry against dissidents. The state relied on psychiatry in two sorts of cases. First, where a dissident had had some psychiatric history, however minor; second, where the dissent might, if charged in court, attract Western publicity. In Grigorenko's case both were true. As a distinguished soldier, he would make good copy and he had been in the Serbsky earlier, in 1964, again for political reasons.

The diagnosis usually used on dissidents was schizophrenia, though some were also labelled 'paranoid personalities'. Once diagnosed, dissidents were sentenced to indefinite spells in special hospitals where the conditions were much like prison. Only when the doctors declared them cured could they be released. Sending sane men to psychiatric hospitals was seen as one more proof of the basic wickedness of the 'Evil Empire'. The Soviet Union denied rights to religious groups, to Jews, and policed its own citizens much as Orwell had predicted in *1984*.

Bloch and Reddaway were always careful. They tried not to sensationalize. They did not suggest that the Soviet Union was the only country in which psychiatry was abused. Their first sentence noted, 'The nature of psychiatry is such that the potential for its improper use is greater than in any other field of medicine.' They did not allege that huge numbers of people were involved. They were always scrupulous about what they did not know. In both these books, they gave lists of dissenters who had been 'abused'. In 1977, the list comprised 210 people; in 1984, it comprised 346. Amnesty also pointed out (1980) how often small acts of protest were enough to 'earn' a diagnosis. They cited cases where someone made religious artifacts (Valeriya Makeyeva), gave song recitals (Pyotr Starchik) and lowered the Soviet flag in Lithuania (Egidius Ionatis).

These accusations finally forced the World Psychiatric Association to take note. Much of the debate at the Honolulu Congress in 1977 centred round this. In 1982, in the run up to the 1983 Vienna Congress, there was increasing pressure to mount some form of inquiry into Soviet practice. The American Psychiatric Association and the Royal College of Psychiatry were the prime movers in that. By 1983 the choice for the Soviet Union was to withdraw or face a debate on political abuse where they risked being censured. It was, however, a close-run thing for many psychiatrists: clearly many felt it was disloyal to question the methods of fellow doctors.

Bloch and Reddaway, like most Western critics, were obliged to write from the outside, relying for information mostly on ex-patients and psychiatrists who had emigrated. Perhaps because of that they tended to divide Soviet psychiatry into a large body of innocents and a few servile devils who did the KGB's dirty work.

The issue became so emotive that one could suggest the Soviet reaction was itself rather neurotic. They slammed the door shut on any reasonable inquiry. The subject was taboo. In 1985, for my film *Forgotten Millions*, which looked at health care round the world, I contacted a Bulgarian psychiatrist, Dr Jablensky, at the World Health Organization. He recommended I write to Dr Vartanyan. I did so and stressed I wasn't interested only in the dissident issue. I never got an answer. An English psychiatrist, Dr Paul Calloway, whom I met in the Soviet Union told me that when he had finally plucked up the courage to raise the issue of political abuse, it had been made clear to him that he had trespassed badly. Invitations were withdrawn; he was told he couldn't meet people. The whole climate surrounding his exchange visits changed radically.

The Soviets remain uncomfortable about the criticisms. At my first meeting with Dr Vartanyan, for example, he criticized how vitriolic Western journalists always were. Dr Potapov, the Russian Minister of Health, agreed to talk to me, for 'unlike most Western journalists, you are not an extremist'. I'm not sure how I gave that useful impression. I talked to Dr Kosirev who was in charge of the Belgrade Hospital to which Grigorenko was released from special hospital. Dr Kosirev specified that Grigorenko was only under his charge for four months but, during those four months, 'I was constantly under siege from the press, especially *Die Stern*.' *Die Stern* offended Kosirev terribly because it published vicious texts about him and a villainous-looking photograph of him. Yet Kosirev insisted he had nothing to do with committing Grigorenko and just wanted to get him out of his hospital as soon as possible. He was co-operating with Mrs Grigorenko to achieve that, he claims. At the time, he did not think Grigorenko was well. He was suffering from arteriosclerosis at least. The injustice of the Western press angered Kosirev.

Sluggish schizophrenia

One of the reasons for Soviet psychiatry's defensiveness was the controversy surrounding 'sluggish schizophrenia'. In a study carried out in 1969, it was found that American and Soviet psychiatrists both tended to diagnose schizophrenia more widely than their colleagues in other parts of the world (Wing 1977). In the Soviet case, one reason for that was the concept of 'sluggish' schizophrenia. Those who suffered from sluggish schizophrenia didn't show extreme signs of frenzy, withdrawal, or hallucinations. Their symptoms were extremely subtle and, sometimes, could only be detected by an equally subtle psychiatrist. Snezhnevsky, longtime director of the Moscow Institute of Psychiatry, said that in the case of sluggish schizophrenia, many of the symptoms would resemble neurotic ones. Some patients would become hypochrondriacs; others paranoid. At times, the patient might even appear well. Paranoid sluggish schizophrenics tended to exaggerate their own importance and to trumpet grandiose ideas. They also tended to offer the world marvellous new ideas.

The diagnosis of sluggish schizophrenia was, in itself, controversial. Szasz (1972) had warned against psychiatry's tendency to spawn endless symptoms of schizophrenia. Snezhnevky had developed the ideas before there was a controversy about dissidents but they turned out to be very useful in the Soviet context. Dissidents did often want to reform the system and to claim that they had the personal vision to do it. They were exhibiting the textbook symptoms of sluggish schizophrenia. The rest of the world never accepted this Soviet diagnosis, always suspecting that it was too convenient for them to be true.

Strangely, two leading human rights activists themselves seem to accept that some of those who dissented were a little odd. Andrei Sakharov noted that, in his experience, many of those who contacted him 'were not mentally stable'.

Podrabinek himself admitted that there was a paradox:

A paradoxical situation arises. There are cases when truly mentally ill people accused of political crimes end up in psychiatric hospitals, that is people who are really acutely ill with delusions. But their delusions have an anti-Soviet colouring. They don't present a danger to anyone . . . obviously people don't laugh at them because they know they're ill and have delusions with a political colouring . . . they're not in anyone's way. But the state reacts in a very touchy way to these ideas, even when they are delusions. Obviously the state realizes the weakness of its regime and its structures, as they're even afraid of the delusions of mentally ill people. We're not even talking of healthy people who express political views. They're even more scared of them.

Both these activists have condemned the use of psychiatry for repression. Podrabinek commented in the IAPUP Bulletin (Dec. 1988) that Sakharov's remarks caused 'desperation and anger.' But these are intriguing remarks.

From the Western view, there are three crucial questions about current psychiatric practice in the USSR:

1. Are there still dissident patients either in ordinary or special hospitals?

2. When are such patients likely to be released and how will their release be handled?

3. Are the Soviet authorities still putting dissident patients inside?

Dissidents still inside

Since 1986, a considerable number of patients who had committed anti-Soviet acts and were held in psychiatric hospitals have been released. The International Association Against the Political Use of Psychiatry believes that many patients have been freed.

There still remain a number of dissident patients who are held inside. There are a variety of Western organizations that publish lists of such patients. These include Amnesty, IAPUP (International Association Against the Political Use of Psychiatry), the Helsinki Watch. According to Amnesty there are 27 people left on their list; according to IAPUP, there are over 200 detained; according to the Helsinki Watch committee, there are some 216 on the list. It is almost certain that there are less than 500 cases of political dissidents still detained.

Many are in special hospitals and, as I shall argue in Chapter Six, the conditions in special hospitals are particularly gruelling.

The Soviet Union has made a commitment to release all political prisoners but, technically, the dissident patients aren't seen as political prisoners. They are seen as sick and in need of treatment. Many of them have been in hospital now for long periods of time like Valery Gromov who wanted to found a people's peasant party and was unwise enough to inform Brezhnev of his plans. Gromov has been detained since 1974 though the authorities say he was convicted for trying to murder his wife. Stomatislav Sudakov has been in special hospitals most of the time since 1974. There are some people on the Amnesty list who are alleged to have been in since the late 1960s.

However unjust their original detention, however sane they originally were, it won't be easy for them to adapt to coming out of hospital. They will need rehabilitation.

When I was filming, a group of twenty American psychiatrists were due to visit the Soviet Union in order to examine about 150 persons whom the West sees as political patients. Under the terms of the agreement worked out between the State Department in Washington, the USSR Foreign Ministry and the Ministry of Health, once a list of patients to be interviewed was agreed, neither side could deviate from it. The Soviets hoped to convince their American colleagues that many of those on this list were in the words of Professor Vartanyan 'nothing to do with political abuse or protests. 40 per cent are criminals, killers, etc etc.' Clever criminals, I was told, tried to dupe Western organizations into adopting them as worthy dissidents. The Americans were given the right to interview the patients. The Soviets believed they would, as good fellow psychiatrists, recognize how fair most of the diagnoses were.

In organizing this visit, the Americans were remarkably secretive. They wouldn't announce what psychiatrists were going or what other experts were accompanying them. In late November 1988 in Moscow, I ran into the advance party who had been sent to negotiate the conditions for the visit. I was returning to the Rossya Hotel when I overheard an American voice saying, 'Goodnight Dr Churkin, I'm sure we'll be able to finish our work.'

Dr Churkin is in charge of psychiatry at the USSR Ministry of Health.

I waited in the lobby for them. When they walked in I asked if they were a party of American psychiatrists. I wasn't aggressive for I had every reason to get them to co-operate with me. They reacted like hunted deer. They looked shocked to have been found. They refused to be interviewed; they refused to say just what they were doing in Moscow and, most bizarre of all, they refused to even give me their names. Their rather ridiculously secretive behaviour illustrates how politically sensitive this whole area is.

Release and rehabilitation

The Soviet authorities won't give any firm commitment on when they will release all dissident patients. Since they don't acknowledge there ever was a policy of detaining dissidents in psychiatric hospitals, it's just a question of when the doctors decide they are cured. The fate of Belov doesn't augur well. He has had little useful help offered. That suggests that it will be important to press for a better deal for patients when they are let out.

Is political abuse still continuing?

This third area has been the most positive. Under glasnost it is possible to speak freely and suggest reforms. People just don't get in trouble as before though there are still occasional cases like that of Alexander Ponomarenko, a member of the Democratic Union who in 1988 was interned in Moscow's 13th Hospital at the request of his mother after she had been visited by the KGB. Another contentious case is that of Anatoly Zhuk who refused to serve in the army. As part of the run up for the 1991 Human Rights Conference Soviet law may change so that anti-Soviet activities would no longer be a crime.

Podrabinek doesn't have much faith in the reforms. He argues that the basic structures that allowed the abuse of psychiatry to take place remain 'and the legal system and the state's attitudes to dissidents haven't changed'.

Nevertheless, Podrabinek had to admit that there had been no cases of people being sent to special hospital for political reasons during the last two years. I asked him if he knew of cases of people being sent to ordinary hospitals. He said he did know of such cases, yes, 'but they are put in hospital and then released. I know of three or four cases this year.' He added cautiously that his concern now was much more to get those who were still inside released.

In an address at the Woodrow Wilson Centre in November 1988 Andrei Sakharov, the physicist who has been such a champion of human rights in the USSR, made some interesting remarks. He condemned the use of psychiatry as 'a tool of political repression and a means of defending the political system'. But he was not sure that political cases had been the numerically greatest abuse. Like Burlatsky, he suggested that perhaps, 'Most victims of psychiatric abuse were people who came into conflict with their superiors and were deemed to be too aggressive in pressing their often legitimate complaints.' Sakharov was more optimistic than Podrabinek. He told his American audience: 'Half a year ago regulations were passed that formally curbed psychiatric abuses for such purposes. Again, I have no exhaustive comprehensive data to support any point of view but there is a widespread feeling that so far the regulations have had no effect. I think such a view is too extreme and that the regulations do work to some extent and have been instrumental in causing a change for the better.'

One of the cases that Podrabinek raised and which certainly illustrated improvement, was that of Vladimir P, which happened in 1988. He was a medical student who wanted to foster better international relations. Rather than beaver away at this worthy aim through official channels, he set off for the American embassy. There had been a bomb scare the week before. The Soviet police guarding the Embassy were suspicious and called in the militia. Vladimir P was taken off to hospital. His family were not told where he was. A commission of two psychiatrists rather than the regular three, declared Vladimir P insane and detained him. His family eventually learned what had happened to him and, within fourteen days, he was released. The really interesting aspect of the case was that it was reported in the press in *Moscow News*. The paper questioned how the authorities had tackled the whole case. Their exposé helped get Vladimir P released and, much like a Western paper that had pulled off such a coup, *Moscow News* trumpeted its part in winning him his freedom.

Podrabinek may be sceptical but he is scrupulously fair. He acknowledged that he was not being harassed now. He was still exiled from Moscow but he was able to publish his *Express Khronika* which took a critical view of current events. When I went to see Podrabinek, he was being visited by the Moscow correspondent of *US News and World Report*. There was nothing clandestine about it. All this openness is strikingly new – and encouraging.

But, as I shall show, psychiatrists still panic at the least mention of politics. My first glimpse of that was in the All Union Centre for Psychiatric Research in Moscow. On the acute ward, I met a slightly vague young man called Sergei Sokov. Sokov seemed rather shy. He had been very interested in philosophy since he was sixteen, had read widely and eventually hallucinated that the KGB was following him. Neither he nor his psychiatrists suggested that he had ever done anything politically. Sokov was said to be in remission after a bad bout of the 'third or fourth order of psychosis'. Not merely was his schizophrenia sluggish but he suffered from 'imperative hallucinations'. Sokov seemed happy to appear on film. He talked a little English and I arranged to film him when we returned to the hospital. The doctors intervened to say they had not agreed to this. They then said pointedly that Sokov was now well enough to go home on week-end leaves. I suggested that we could film him both in the hospital and at home. This would show how it was possible for patients to come and go between the two. Sokov agreed to this. Sokov seemed amiable and rather woolly, far more a dreamer than a dissident. The doctors told me that he said aliens from outer space instructed him to immerse himself in philosophical ideas. Sokov, however, didn't accept this verdict. He did look a little confused but, in a small stubborn way, insisted he had been interested in these ideas since he was a teenager.

When I returned to the hospital to film, he wasn't there. He had changed his mind I was told, by the staff. It was to be the first of many obstructions.

At various points in this book, as they happened in various institutions, I have logged the problems there were in securing interviews and the dramas that occurred when interviews went wrong from the Soviet point of view. Dr Egorov had promised me full access and urged Western psychiatrists to accept 'we have no secrets'. But I came across many exceptions. It's important to be fair to the Soviets. Psychiatric institutions all over the world tend to be guarded. I have been, over the years, denied permission to film in Broadmoor and in the emergency clinic of the Maudsley. But in the Soviet Union, the nervousness nearly always occurred when there was fear a patient might turn out to have a political tinge. I found it understandable but irritating. More seriously, it made me see how hard it must be to change the reflexes of Soviet psychiatry.

When I raised the question of whether there had been a systematic policy of abuse, I didn't expect to get an abject, apologetic 'yes'. But I did expect a certain degree of 'give'. There was little sign of that, however.

The following psychiatrists denied there had ever been such malpractice: Dr G. Morosov of the Serbsky, Dr Vartanyan of the USSR Academy of Medical Sciences, Dr V. Egorov, head of psychiatry and narcology at the USSR Ministry of Health, Dr A. Potapov, who was head of psychiatry at Tomsk before he became the Minister of Health of the Russian Federation, Professor Modest Kabanov of the Bechterev Institute in Leningrad. The most eloquent and perhaps amusing denial came from Professor Zharikov who is the new President of the Association of Soviet Psychiatrists. Zharikov alleged that 'these dissidents, they did it for the money and for their popularity'. He waved his arms upwards for emphasis.

Few people in the West are likely to be convinced by these denials, however eloquent, and I am not. There clearly was abuse and, clearly too, a number of normal people were put away in psychiatric hospitals. In other cases, people who were mildly disturbed but had unorthodox views were treated with quite unnecessary harshness. Many were sent like Grigorenko to a special top-security hospital when there was no evidence that they were a danger. At the time he was over seventy!

The general line taken by Soviet psychiatrists is that there may well have been individual mistakes, as with Medvedev. Dr Zharikov said that it was possible that there had even been some abuses because of the criminal irresponsibility and negligence of some doctors. Some of these cases could have been political. Dr Egorov at the Ministry of Health did acknowledge that there were 'people who were put in hospital who had ideas that were contrary to the prevailing ideology. And this was seen as one sign of their mental illness. But the extent to which they were ill is a more complicated matter.' Dr Egorov was willing to concede that by today's standards, the treatment they received was harsh. 'There were cases of hospitalization which were not necessary but they occurred,' he said. 'There were cases of excessive supervision by psychiatrists.' He came closer than any other official to admitting consistent errors but even he rejected the idea that this added up to abuse. The unwillingness of Soviet doctors to actually admit there was, if not a policy of abuse, a regular set of errors, is striking.

In many areas of Soviet life, the State is now being severely criticized. Stalin's policies and Brezhnev's 'period of stagnation' led to individual injustices. Citizens were denied many rights to which, in theory, they were entitled. The press has exposed corruption and incompetence. I picked up rumours that some psychiatrists were being investigated for corruption. In such circumstances, it's possible to understand why psychiatrists should be wary, but these changes also present an opportunity for reassessing the past role of psychiatry.

In the changing political situation of the Soviet Union, it would be possible for psychiatrists to suggest that they had been put under intolerable political pressure and that this led to the abuse. They could point the finger at a political system which has now been heavily criticized. They could joke that perhaps the man with the greatest 'reformist delusions' is Gorbachev. They have taken none of these steps.

This suggests that the roots of the abuse were more complex than Western critics allowed. After all, if the psychiatrists were just creatures of the Kremlin, why not denounce the mistakes of the past as has happened in many areas of Soviet life. Let self-criticism, that new orthodoxy, bloom. I have already suggested it is too simplistic to see the abuse in terms of politicians ordering doctors to commit particular individuals. Bloch and Reddaway themselves cite many instances of doctors who refused to commit, like Professor Detengof, who wouldn't commit Grigorenko, and Dr Shostakovitch, who could not pinpoint any acute psychological disorder in Medvedev while he was in Kaluga. I want to suggest that the psychiatrists find it hard to admit there was abuse not just because that would be embarrassing but because they have rationalized their behaviour away. Segal (1976) claimed that psychiatrists were bureaucratic, inclined to trust those in authority and to doubt anyone who behaved in an unconventional manner. It wasn't hard for them to convince themselves that dissidents were sick. Many Soviet texts, like *The Pictorial Language of Schizophrenics*, convey a very unflattering picture of the patient. He isn't just ill but sloppy, untidy, vain, deformed, a hopeless human mess. As a result, Soviet psychiatrists still bring to their patients a very authoritarian attitude. Trust the doctor. He, or she, knows everything. Patients should be grateful to have beds, how dare they want rights? With such a low opinion of patients, it doesn't require Machiavellian careerist doctors to mistreat patients for love of the Kremlin.

Naturally, Soviet psychiatrists would prefer to avoid the embarrassment of admitting there were mistakes. Such an admission would invite questions about the whole practice of Soviet psychiatry – not just the treatment of dissidents. Psychiatrists are far too insecure in the present changing circumstances to welcome that.

But for the West too, it's easier not to ask whether the political abuse was a special form of general abuse. Bloch and Reddaway subtitled *Soviet Psychiatric Abuse* 'the shadow over world psychiatry'. But there are many other shadows, too, some of which have caused more suffering to more people than even the Soviet one. There have been allegations of abuse of patients in Britain, the USA, Japan, Holland, Norway, West Germany and in less developed countries like India and Egypt. In 1984, the year *Soviet Psychiatric Abuse* appeared, the Japanese press revealed that 221 patients had died in Utsonomiya Hospital in the previous three years in mysterious circumstances. Surely as much of a shadow as anything in the Serbsky! But it suited some Western commentators to act as if the Soviet situation was unique. To link political abuse to the ordinary abuse patients can suffer everywhere is to question the particular evil of the Soviet situation. Yet in every culture, there is fear of mental illness and prejudice against the mentally ill. The Soviet Union is typical in that. Fear and prejudice make it easy for psychiatrists to exercise great power.

Psychiatry invites abuse for its history is intimately linked to the need for social control in industrialized countries. Historians like Scull (1983) have argued that the rise of psychiatry coincided with the Industrial Revolution. Medicine, which was gaining greatly in scientific prestige in the nineteenth century, offered society the chance to control and care for rebels, misfits and the inadequate. To place them in asylums where they might be cured also looked humane, much nicer than locking them up in prisons.

The struggle to create a proper set of legal safeguards to balance these powers wasn't easy for Western lawyers. The more conformist the society the less motivation it has to give patients any rights. In Japan, many of the 330,000 people who ended up detained were people who didn't fit into the pattern of the Japanese economic miracle. It took years of exposure of terrible abuses and much international pressure to create better laws. In Britain, prejudice has become more of a problem than conformity. Far more young blacks are diagnosed as schizophrenic than statistically expected. It's not poor genes but rich cultural differences. White and Indian doctors interpret the loud, very energetic behaviour of West Indians as aggressive and crazy. It's not the way the British behave so it must be schizophrenia. High-spirited fun becomes florid sickness. The norm of one culture is the abnormal of another (Rack 1982).

When I put it to Dr Bloch that patients in many cultures had been unjustly detained, he agreed. He accepted, too, that an excessive number of blacks had been diagnosed schizophrenic in the UK. 'But that problem can be discussed freely,' he said. For him that seemed to prove abuse here was radically different from abuse in the Soviet Union.

But some Western academics are beginning to inquire into this area. Parchomenko (1986) in a study of Soviet images of dissidence noted that this whole area was neglected. He concluded that Soviet officials had an image of dissidents which was 'greatly distorted, stereotypic, tending to caricature but nevertheless held with a measure of conviction . . .' (p. 172). Like Segal, Parchomenko suggests we need a more sophisticated account than pure cynicism or evil. This is not to accept what Soviet psychiatry did but to acknowledge the complexity of the issue.

Psychiatric abuse is an international problem. One particular form thrived in the Soviet Union and was seized on by the West as proof of the iniquity of Communism. The West was only interested in political abuse. But many apolitical patients suffered poor and unjust treatment too, a situation which made political abuse easier. In looking at the treatment of ordinary patients in the next two chapters, I shall outline some of these non-political abuses. Western critics hardly commented on them. It was cosier not to underline the ways in which Soviet and Western psychiatry could be similar.

4

Community Care: The Dispensaire *System*

Sergei Belov sees his local *dispensaire* as an outpost of the militia. Though he is now free, he still has to report there every month. The *dispensaire* is part of the state's controlling apparatus. For many patients, going to the *dispensaire* is a happier experience, but it's not hard to see why Belov feels embittered by it.

In the sixties, anti-psychiatrists argued that psychiatry was a therapeutic fraud. It pretended to offer care and cure; in fact, it offered little care and a great deal of control. R. D. Laing (1972) and Thomas Szasz in *The Manufacture of Madness* (1972) would have seen in the *dispensaire* system a perfect illustration of their thesis. Unlike Bloch and Reddaway, Laing and Szasz both claimed that all psychiatry was political and repressive. The state was trying to monitor its misfits by labelling them mad. Though most *dispensaire* patients are apolitical and many say they are helped, the structure of the system shows with exceptional clarity how all psychiatry can be used for social control. Yet ironically, the *dispensaire* system could also be seen as a model example of community care.

If a Soviet citizen is ill, he or she generally goes to the local poliklinik. The poliklinik is a general health centre. Its doctors usually have no psychiatric qualification. Individuals with psychiatric or psychological difficulties are sent to the *dispensaire*. Many people told me that if they felt distressed, they would seek private help. Coming under the *dispensaire* was a frightening prospect. A few individuals seek help freely but because there are so few voluntary patients, it's more usual for patients to be referred. Families, neighbours and work colleagues often insist individuals get treatment. Vladimir, a man of fifty, alleged, 'My wife and mother-in-law informed on me.' Fyodor

Burlatsky, co-chair of the Commission on Human Rights, said that they had received far more complaints from those whose families had tried to get them committed and those 'who had been sent for psychiatric treatment by their bosses' than from political cases. Burlatsky described a typical case. A worker would criticize their boss and find themselves 'accused of social delusions'. Even now, people are referred for unconventional or eccentric behaviour.

On any one day, about 150 to 200 patients come to the 14th *dispensaire* in Moscow which has 4,885 patients on its register. Very few are voluntary patients, though many are perfectly glad to seek treatment. With some, the *dispensaire* doesn't mind if they turn up or they don't. Others know that they will be in trouble if they don't report in. It might mean being hauled off to hospital. Most *dispensaire* patients have conventional psychiatric problems. They're depressed or schizophrenic or in conflict with their families. Some abuse the system. A few patients confessed they came because it allowed them to avoid work.

The *dispensaire* system was set up in order to provide ordinary people with something they had been denied before the 1917 Revolution – decent health care. During the civil war that followed, the Soviet Union was ravaged by typhus. The newsreels of the time covered the epidemic and the terrible suffering it caused. Millions died. One newsreel highlighted the image of a skeletal horse in the snow which was a bag of bones. The need to fight the epidemic made the Bolshevik government focus on the need for health care for ordinary people.

In 1921, the government started a system of *dispensaires*. The French word has been used to describe them from the start. Newsreel footage exists of a congress of Moscow doctors who heard, and applauded, the setting up of such a system. They were told that now that they had conquered the epidemic, they must produce positive good health. Only a healthy population would be fit to carry out the task of the Revolution. *Dispensaires*, by the 1950s, concentrated on psychiatry alone: general medicine relied on the polikliniks.

The 14th *dispensaire* is housed in what used to be a rich merchant's house on Chekhov Street. The entrance is rather grand. A marble staircase leads to a landing with a fine balustrade: the doors are large and emblazoned with elaborate designs. On the second floor, there is a day hospital; on the first floor rooms for hypnosis, physiotherapy and sleep therapy. The ground floor has a suite for acupuncture and an outpatient clinic. In an annexe, there's a space for work therapy and, at the moment, a room in the basement houses the Moscow Psychotherapy Unit. As this list shows, treatments strange in the West aren't strange at all in the USSR.

The Chekhov Street house is the kind the Russian bourgeoisie would have given balls in. Today, however, the entrance is piled with builders' rubbish. In many hospitals, perestroika has meant that they are finally getting some maintenance, a 'remonte', from the French word *remonter*. The remonte is not wholly good. The building's fine marble floor is being covered with cheap and uncheerful lino.

The 14th *dispensaire* is in central Moscow. Just round the corner is Pushkin Square, one of Moscow's most historic squares dominated by a statue of the poet Pushkin and by an ornate fountain. A number of major Soviet institutions have offices in the square including the newspapers *Isvestia, Moscow News* and *Moscow Pravda*. The city's largest cinema is there too and there are also a few cafés including one which was a haunt for dubious right-wingers. Despite its central location, the *dispensaire* doesn't face the typical city centre problems of the West. The most notorious excesses in Pushkin Square can't hope to rival Piccadilly or Times Square. No drunks, no drug dealing, no rent boys.

Few of the patients I talked to in the *dispensaire* denied that they had serious problems.

Of the twelve patients I talked to eleven were totally apolitical. They suffered from depression, schizophrenia or generally a sense of inadequacy. The director, Dr Passer, said that they had many cases of family conflict.

Sasha was a typical example. He was a gangly young man who worked as a cook when he was well. Dr Passer explained his schizophrenia had upset his family. Sasha's mother was at her wits' end. Dr Passer talked to him affectionately but very patronizingly. She repeatedly said to Sasha that he was a good nice boy but ill and irritating. Sasha accepted this with a certain resignation and didn't argue back.

Dr Passer was clearly annoyed by the fecklessness of some of her charges. A smartly dressed man moaned that he was a musician and too tense to work. Dr Passer said that he was too idle and made too many demands on his family. One patient, a rumbustious man in his sixties smiled as he said that his family was 60 per cent understanding. You couldn't expect more. The big difficulty had been giving up drink because he had lost all his friends.

There was little tension in the *dispensaire* even though some patients were clearly disturbed. A schizophrenic girl from Central Asia said with a certain splendid vacantness, 'I like it here. The work is easy. I am beautiful.'

Before the current controversies about dissidents, the *dispensaire* system had a good press which stressed its caring role. The controlling role was hardly noticed. As late as 1976 Holland (1976), concluded that in many ways the Soviet system offered better health care than a capitalist system that would never invest as much in medicine. She called the *dispensaires* 'excellent community-based centres'.

Few of the treatments on offer are energetic. In the day hospital, patients sit, either in the corridor or in a large room where they can watch television. Some seem perfectly well. One woman was knitting meticulously. The rumbustious man explained that it was quite nice to come here. The musician added that he had been helped by the doctors. He said he soon hoped to be playing again. Perhaps he'd heard the doctor's complaints about his laziness. In the afternoon, the musician went to have sleep therapy for his appalling insomnia. One of the cures on offer is what the doctors there call 'electro sleep'. Patients lie down and leather thongs are put over their eyes. Then they are attached to a small machine which gives them a tiny burst of electricity, about 2 volts. The procedure looks sinister but the patients seemed to enjoy it. The musician said this was a very relaxing form of sleep. Even children are given it.

The main treatment room also had in it a 'magnetomachine' which wasn't being used. Patients could be given the benefit of having magnets waved over them. I joked to the doctor that this seemed like Mesmer. Back in the 1780s, Mesmer took Paris and Vienna by storm when he claimed to cure patients by using magnetism. The French king, Louis XVI, set up a commission which eventually proved Mesmer was a fraud and that he got his successes by suggestion. But Dr Passer didn't seem to know the historical reference.

The slightly mystical nature of some of the treatment is most evident in group hypnosis. There's a special room with ten couches in it. I watched one of the therapists put a group to sleep, telling them to relax, forget about their tensions, forget about their bodies, forget . . . She chanted the instructions like a mantra.

Many of these patients suffered from chronic anxiety. Some were worried that perestroika would change their working lives. It was exotic and a little touching to watch these sober-seeming middle-aged men and women drift into relaxation, all together. One man started to snore, all tension gone. The hypnotist said that for many problems, this technique worked well. She had even used hypnosis with couples who had marital troubles. Some Soviet research argues the technique works well. The hypnosis room was the only place where I saw a picture of Freud. He beamed down, appropriately, since he had used hypnosis and suggestion before inventing psychoanalysis.

On the ground floor there's a room dedicated to acupuncture. The walls are lined with acupuncture charts including a vastly blown up map of the ear. The acupuncturist explained that she used a French technique which linked parts of the ear to various problems. She giggled when she pointed out those parts to needle for marital problems. She was treating a patient with a weight problem. Even the acupuncturist suffered from lack of equipment. On my first visit, she said she did electro-acupuncture too. When I returned to film and requested a demonstration, she became embarrassed. She hadn't used the electro-acupuncture equipment for eighteen months, she admitted, because she didn't have the batteries needed to make it function. It was a pity, she sniped, that the West was so interested in the problems of dissidents and never bothered with the real problems of ordinary patients. Since I was there with a film crew, we were able to supply her with batteries.

Shortages also mean that the *dispensaire* doesn't do ECT. Dr Passer explained that they were a little frightened of ECT but now they had finally ordered a machine.

The *dispensaire* seems to make an effort to inform patients about their medication. A shabby noticeboard has sample packs of the drugs. The accompanying legends reveal what the drugs do and what their after-effects are. Someone had scrawled over the pack of amphetamines 'Joy'. The *dispensaire* gives depot phenothiazines (a drug for schizophrenics) and checks that patients do take their drugs. Those on the register have to take the drugs they are prescribed.

In many Soviet hospitals, there are rumours that drugs are stolen. There is a lucrative black market so it's not strange that the security surrounding drugs is strict. Everywhere I was allowed in, I tried to make sure that there weren't isolation or punishment cells as one of the allegations made by Bloch and Reddaway is that these are used to discipline patients. In the *dispensaire*, there was a barred entrance to a very dark-looking space. At last, I'd found a cage! It turned out that they kept most of their drugs there, safely locked away.

There are perfectly conventional treatments, too, at the *dispensaire*. The girl who declared herself to be beautiful was in a group of eight who were doing work therapy which consisted of sticking labels on to lipstick canisters. All the others in that group were elderly. In the day hospital, two patients were sleeping in a small dormitory. They didn't seem to be receiving any treatment. On our second visit, a middle-aged man was on a drip getting intravenous antidepressants.

The *dispensaire*'s job is also to monitor patients who are on the register at home. In theory, this is the kind of after-care that should be beneficial. Families can, and often do, ring up when someone is deteriorating. Dr Passer explained that they were often able to prevent acute episodes by knowing when to hospitalize patients and bring them in for treatment or, in some cases, admit them to hospital. One of the ways of checking is through frequent home visits.

I went with one doctor to see a young patient who was

suffering from progressively worsening schizophrenia. We set off in the *dispensaire* ambulance. It is very basic and carries no emergency kit at all. We got out and, while we went up to the eighth floor, the ambulance waited for the doctor. It's hard to imagine that neighbours wouldn't start to gossip about the reason for the ambulance waiting outside for twenty minutes.

On the eighth floor, a short plump woman greeted us but not with any great relief. The doctor went in to talk to her son. The mother spoke English and explained that she really didn't have much faith in the care offered. It was just drugs and the drugs hadn't helped her son much. Sadly, he was her only son.

It wasn't wholly clear why the visit was necessary. The son seemed perfectly calm, if a little surly. The doctor asked him how he was, chatted for about five minutes and then wrote out a prescription. The doctor talked to the grandmother but not the mother. Once we were outside, the doctor said that the patient would never improve. He couldn't work and was getting, at the age of twenty, an invalidity pension. He would go downhill from now on. The doctor foresaw that in a few years he would be in hospital.

In most towns, the *dispensaire* is in a separate setting well away from the hospital. In Kaluga, a town 180 kilometres outside Moscow which has a large and well-known hospital, a different system has been tried. The *dispensaire* is actually inside the hospital. This allows patients to be seen by the same doctor whether they are receiving outpatient or inpatient care. The director of the Kaluga Hospital, Dr Lifschitz, argued that this made it easier to know when to admit patients and also easier to keep a check on them when they were released.

In many ways, the *dispensaire* provides accessible, and good, care. But this hasn't created tolerance. The service has to battle with the prejudices of society against mental patients which are as pronounced in the Soviet Union as elsewhere. I couldn't track down any Soviet studies of attitudes to mental illness but nearly every doctor I talked to bemoaned the fact that the public was hostile. In Leningrad, Dr Khashkarov of the Bechterev said that they had problems both with industry and even with museums when they wanted to arrange outings. Many patients complained that if they were on the register and their places of work knew about it, they were discriminated against. Dr Passer said that they tried to keep the information that someone was on the register confidential. When they went to visit someone in their home, they didn't tell neighbours. They did not tell factories or offices that someone employed by them was on the register because 'We want to see that inmates don't lose their jobs. But there is prejudice in organizations.' Dr Passer's concern seemed sincere to my colleagues who were adept at picking up signs of liberalism. They noted that Dr Passer had some progressive trophies. Her mantelpiece sported a picture of Vyssotsky, a very popular dissident singer during the Brezhnev era. Anyone who displayed that was bound to have good instincts. Dr Passer said that they tried to resist pinning a diagnosis of schizophrenia on someone. 'We like to delay doing that.' The consequences of being so diagnosed could be severe.

Yet the very structure of the register and the obligations it imposes on the doctors mean that the information can't be kept that confidential. There is, moreover, a Soviet tradition not of citizens 'informing' against each other but of keeping others up to scratch.

In every part of the Soviet Union, the *dispensaires* are responsible for administering the register. They decide who goes on the register and who goes off it. The new law has made their task more complicated since there is now some pressure to reduce the numbers of people on the register. Dr Passer explained that they had 4,885 people on the list. It had been 5,800 recently. They had, as a result of the new law, been reviewing their register. They had released 885 patients from the list. But their criteria were very stringent. A schizophrenic had to have been in remission for five years. Dr Passer added that she tried to explain to those on the register why it wasn't possible to free them. Most accepted the decision but there were a small number who continued to be dissatisfied. In a few cases, they had been violent. She said that one man had threatened her with a hammer. Another colleague said she had been attacked with an axe. Quite often psychiatrists mentioned the dangers of their trade. One who works in the *dispensaire* had been badly injured when the friends of a patient stabbed him in the neck.

The 14th *dispensaire* seemed a benign if rather nannying institution until I said that I wanted to interview a fat, bearded patient in the day hospital. I had been assured that I could interview anyone I wanted. The young doctor in charge of the day hospital told me that I shouldn't really talk to this particular patient. I repeated the assurances made to me and was told this patient was very disturbed and aggressive. He wouldn't make a nice interview. The patient looked sullen and was walking restlessly up and down the corridor. I imagined that the doctor knew that he was the kind of patient who was angry and would be critical. But, as what happened shows, there was more to it than that.

Ephraim sat heavily down on the sofa. Six other patients stayed in the room, as did the doctor. It was the only instance in the *dispensaire* when an interview was supervised. Ephraim began by saying that he did not like being on the register. His response to it was 'negative. I'm treated like a black in America.'

I asked him if he felt he had suffered as a result. 'Yes, I have suffered,' he concluded weightily. He then paused for a long while. 'Yes, I have suffered since 1978 when I went to the American embassy to make inquiries about how to emigrate to Israel. I'm of Jewish nationality.' He then settled back to see how everyone absorbed this.

I asked him if he thought he would be allowed to emigrate when his treatment was finished. Ephraim said he would like to emigrate, 'But I do not think I will be given a chance. They will take revenge on me. Just a few minutes ago that doctor – Nikolai Arkady, I don't know his surname – hissed at me urging me to refuse this interview.' Again Ephraim paused weightily. 'He said he'd cart me off to hospital if I disobeyed.'

At this point, the doctor intervened. Tellingly, he didn't deny the accusation. Fairly softly, he said, 'But you said you've been feeling unwell since 1978. What kind of measures have been applied to you? And how?'

Ephraim ignored these attempts to get him to discuss his symptoms publicly. He alleged that he had been badly treated in a hospital. At which point two patients sitting by the doctor started to chant, 'It's not true. It's not true.' One of these was the musician.

The chant over, the doctor returned to the attack. Ephraim had told him he had been influenced from the outside. The implication was that Ephraim's head buzzed with alien voices. 'What do you feel about them? Did they exercise a kind of remote control over you?'

Ephraim shrugged. 'I don't know.'

'But you told me,' insisted the doctor.

'If I told you why do you ask, then?'

'You told me about being influenced from a distance,' repeated the doctor. 'Tell us about that.'

It was a fairly amazing scene with the doctor badgering the patient to reveal his symptoms to an audience. I couldn't tell whether Ephraim had these symptoms or not. He answered all my questions rationally and appropriately. However, his appearance was scruffy and that of a man who wasn't too comfortable in his body. Lack of grace is not, however, a psychiatric symptom.

After that exchange there didn't seem anything more to ask. Ephraim got up. I asked his name and he gave it in full. Ephraimov Lev Andylyevich. He added his address; flat 40, 27 Planetaya Street.

The doctor then insisted on giving us all Ephraim's clinical details to establish that he really was ill. The story about the Embassy was, he claimed, a fantasy. Ephraim's parents were driven crazy by him. He worked in a boiler-room and constantly irritated all his colleagues who couldn't stand him. He was very childish and, of course, schizophrenic. The very anxious doctor must have spent fifteen minutes giving us confidential clinical details. Then, in the middle of the next interview that was being filmed, Dr Passer appeared. She too was very flustered. She hoped we wouldn't misunderstand the case. He was a sick man, not a dissident. She was clearly shaken by the account she had been given of the scene.

Such scenes and the bitterness that both Ephraim and Belov had displayed mean that it's impossible to see the *dispensaire* as just an uncomplicated health centre providing effective community care.

The Chief Psychiatrist

It was an old Russian tradition that the poor serf could appeal directly to the Tsar. The Tsars often hung boxes out of their palaces into which the people could place petitions. The Tsar held his throne by divine right, and the people could make supplication to him. Where those who suffered injustices once appealed to the Tsar, they can now appeal to the Chief Psychiatrist of Moscow.

In Chapter Two, I explained that the Chief Psychiatrist of various towns is now responsible for running commissions to which patients can appeal. In Moscow, the Chief Psychiatrist has a number of offices in various *dispensaires*. The 14th *dispensaire* is one of the places where there are commission hearings. Ordinary members of the public can also queue to see the Chief Psychiatrist or his deputy twice a week from 2 P.M. to 4 P.M.. People come here with complaints of all sorts about the psychiatric system.

There were only two people waiting to consult the Chief Psychiatrist. One was a middle-aged lady with flat brown hair. She had a pastry-coloured face. She explained that her daughter had had two breakdowns. Then, about a year ago, she had had a third breakdown. To make matters worse she had had severe inflammation of the foot. She had been admitted to hospital and had been there for eleven months. But she wasn't getting any better. She thought her daughter could do better in a research institute. She hoped the Chief Psychiatrist could help.

The second person waiting outside illustrated many of the problems that the *dispensaire* system creates. He was an old man who eventually said he was ninety years old. He was reading *Pravda*. He was bald and wore glasses. For ninety, he seemed very fit but he was rather diffident. It took a little time for him to explain. He wanted to see the Chief Psychiatrist because his neighbours had written to the *dispensaire* to say he was crazy. On the basis of that alone, he had been 'inspected' by *dispensaire* doctors but they had decided not to put his name on the register. The neighbours' accusation and the visit of the doctors had made the people suspicious of him. He now wanted an official letter saying that he was sane. He had come to

request a certificate of sanity. It seemed that only then could
he feel at peace again.

Transmash

Until recently, an apparently successful *dispensaire* system
seemed to exclude the need for other forms of community care.
Slowly, that is changing. Some psychiatrists, like Professor
Alexandrovsky of the Serbsky, realize that it's important to
encourage people who need help to come and seek treatment
of their own free will. He told me, 'Soviet psychiatry is coming
out of the madhouse.' Alexandrovsky's many roles show how
easy it is to be simplistic about Soviet psychiatry. He's Deputy
Director of the Serbsky and, therefore, repressive; he is also
one of the USSR's leading experts on how to handle disasters
and was heavily involved in counselling victims of Chernobyl;
finally, he has been one of the prime movers in a new, and very
unrepressive, facility called Transmash. Transmash is a car and
tractor factory in Moscow. It is in the process of building a
psychological health club for its workers. The club is housed in
a narrow building tucked down a side alley. The only surprise
given the bleak street is that there's a huge Aztec face mask by
the front door. The inside is extraordinary. The walls are lined
with silver metal donated by the factory. The metal has been
cut into thin strips so you feel you're walking along walls of
silver tagliatelle. This intense surreal decor carries on throughout the club. On the first floor is what they call a hypnotarium.
The treatment here is similar to that offered in the 14th
dispensaire but the surroundings are infinitely more stylish.

The workers recline in comfy armchairs. Rather good paintings in the style of Bosch cover the walls. In one corner, a
soothing fountain splashes. To symbolize the fears lurking
inside the mind, there's a montage of bars and devil masks on
the wall. While the hypnotist urges the workers to forget their
bodies, forget their minds, forget their tensions, music plays
too. The whole setting is extremely relaxing.

People come here after work to have a 'mental sauna', as Dr
Alexandrovsky put it. The club also has rooms for psychotherapy, counselling and sleep therapy. Alexandrovsky and his

colleagues at Transmash have also encouraged psychodrama. 'We use it especially with alcoholics,' he said.

On Saturday morning, I went to the club to see drama students do a short play in which a young man goes on the booze. The meeting room downstairs was packed with perhaps 150 people. Some had psychological problems: others were friends of the cast. The drama wasn't subtle. The young boozer's career and marriage are in ruins. His friends desert him. But his trusting wife decides to give him one more chance. Her faith restores him. Result: happiness and cure.

Some of the audience asked: what if the wife hadn't been such a paragon?

The drama students came back. Their next piece was even briefer. The wretched wino entered a restaurant, tried to borrow money from his friends and then made a pass at a girl. His friends left him at once. His wife spurned him since she knew about the pass. Within three minutes, he was back on the bottle. Forever, we were led to believe.

Alexandrovsky conceded that it was melodramatic but the audience enjoyed it. One man who sported the nearest thing to a handlebar moustache I saw in the Soviet Union explained to me that as an alcoholic he had been sent to a special facility where they had to work all the time. It was a kind of drying out centre with hard labour. He had hated it and he had managed to get himself discharged. The so-called therapy hadn't helped him. He came to Transmash not just for the psychodrama but for counselling and relaxation. He said that that had helped him more.

Alexandrovsky stressed that Transmash wasn't unique. There was another such health club at the Zil car factory and, increasingly, there would be more. Such preventive services were very important, especially at a time of social change which many people found confusing and hard to manage.

I have suggested that, in some ways, the *dispensaire* system provided a framework for community care long before community care became a chic concept. The *dispensaires* are well-established neighbourhood centres which offer many services. Their framework makes it possible to identify many of those who need care. Further, Dr Tichonenko, the Chief Psychiatrist of Moscow, claimed the relationship between most *dispensaires* and local hospitals was good.

The *dispensaires* also provide a good basis for aftercare. In the West, one of the perennial problems of psychiatry is that patients get lost in the gaps in the system. They are discharged from hospital and no one knows where they go. Thousands in America, and increasingly in the UK, end up on the streets homeless, helpless and without any care. I didn't see any homeless mentally ill in Moscow, Leningrad and Kaluga. One reason is the *dispensaire* system.

Another reason is that their presence would offend what I can only call social discipline. Dr Egorov of the Ministry of Health stressed the way in which psychiatrists were determined to prevent 'socially dangerous acts' by their patients. Those with psychiatric difficulties of any kind have been strictly controlled. That has made the *dispensaires* the first unit of control and, from what I saw, rather heavy-handed. It hasn't been just politically troublesome patients who suffer. Ordinary patients are also treated in a rather disciplined and sometimes disparaging way. They are often spoken to rather like wayward children. The doctors don't seem to have much concept of creating a 'therapeutic alliance' in which the expert and the sick reach together towards cure. The research done on learned helplessness (Seligman 1975) and on the dangers of institutionalization both suggest that keeping patients 'down' in such a way is likely to delay cure and harm them.

The *dispensaire* system needs to change radically. It needs to adapt to the fact that more patients will be voluntary patients and will not accept the kind of control that's been common practice.

I had planned to end this chapter with a summary of the pros and cons of the *dispensaire* system. Then I remembered one of the odd things that happened during my visit. In the 14th *dispensaire*, there was only one doctor who seemed to be really interested in how psychiatry was organized in Britain. She asked for details of how people were admitted and what safeguards there were in the fabled West. She ran the home visit section and I looked forward to interviewing her on film.

On the day of the filming she wasn't there. Eventually, a little embarrassed, Yelena told me what had happened. 'She's had a breakdown,' Yelena said. 'She's in hospital herself.'

I was sad but not surprised because by then I was beginning to learn that one of the curious facts about Soviet psychiatric hospitals is that they are full of doctors who have been sent there for treatment.

5
Kashenko

No society is very comfortable in dealing with sick doctors. In Britain, research shows that doctors are particularly prone to mental illness, alcoholism and drug taking. Usually, doctors are kept out of ordinary psychiatric hospitals; they're seen privately. One or two private sanatoriums do a nice trade, providing a retreat for medics who can no longer take it.

As I was soon to discover, sick doctors are commonplace in the Soviet Union's psychiatric hospitals. Even more surprising, perhaps, is that they are treated with very little deference. At the Kaluga Hospital I met a plump middle-aged woman who said she was a doctor. She wore a scarf around her head and was working patiently assembling electronic equipment elements for cars. She didn't grumble. At the All Union Centre in Moscow, a woman in her late forties sat on her bed and stared at her rather loud room-mate. 'I used to be a cardiologist,' she said, wrapping her thin shawl round her bony shoulders. She was a specialist but that didn't protect her when she started having breakdowns. But once, they were short of staff in the ward and she had been asked to help decipher an ECG. 'I found I could still do it,' she smiled, but that one moment of skill rediscovered, a moment that was now some years ago, hadn't changed anything. I asked her why she didn't join the other patients on the walks. 'When my husband left me, he took my coat,' she sighed. It was below freezing outside and, without warm clothes, she couldn't go. She explained that the hospital had its problems and couldn't provide a coat. There really were no privileges for doctors.

Both these doctors had accepted that, in reality, they were never going to practise medicine again. The sense of shame at suddenly being a patient is most acute among those who still hope. Anna had been at the Kashenko Hospital in Moscow for three months. Dark haired, about thirty, she sat tensely in an armchair. She said she felt 'very weak' because she had had terrible times in her family. She didn't want to elaborate on those misfortunes. The treatment in the hospital was good but she felt sad. She wanted to resume her work on psychopharmacology. She was in the middle of her thesis on benzodiazepines and that, now, had to be put back. Not for ever, she said. 'Next time I hope you'll talk to me as an expert, not a patient.' She asked me which psychiatrists I had seen and, when I gave her a list, she said she knew of some of them and had attended a conference where Vartanyan spoke. At the end of our conversation, the ward doctor was silent. If it had occurred to him that it might be hard for her to adapt to being a patient, he didn't say.

The doctors got no preferential treatment. Once they were sick, they were patients like any other.

In trying to describe life in the ordinary hospitals, I've drawn on interviews with doctors, with ex-patients and on what I observed in three ordinary hospitals I visited at length – the Kashenko in Moscow, the Bechterev Institute in Leningrad and Kaluga Hospital some 180 miles outside Moscow. I don't claim this chapter is a scientific survey of Soviet hospital life. Rather it is impressionistic and it is as well to remember that all three institutions are well-known and possibly, therefore, better than average. The Kashenko and the Bechterev receive many visitors from abroad; Kaluga Hospital is beginning to make a name for itself as an innovator in work therapy, a topic I cover in Chapter Eight.

Overcrowding

For the majority of patients, the facilities are not that good. Soviet psychiatric hospitals tend to be large and rather Victorian, constructed round long, echoing corridors. Many of the problems they face are familiar. Hospitals are trying to treat patients in poor buildings designed long ago. Many of the buildings are now dilapidated. Many wards are overcrowded.

Frequently, psychiatrists told me they didn't know how they

were going to cope with the increasing number of old people who were going to live longer and become senile. The Soviet family is aping the West, becoming more mobile, less devoted to its elderly. There is a further, specifically Soviet problem. The trade unions provide many retirement homes and, according to some psychiatrists, they are prejudiced against the mentally ill. Sanatoriums for the physically ill exist, but unions have built few for those with psychiatric problems. If families and trade unions aren't coping, the burden is likely to fall on hospitals.

The Kashenko is one of Moscow's oldest hospitals. It was set up by public subscription in 1894 when it cost 1 million gold roubles. Today, there are 2,600 beds. The hospital stretches over 40 acres. In the snow, it looked rather bleak. The entrance to the administration building resembles curiously the entrance to Broadmoor. The hospital has twenty-six wards. I was allowed to visit anywhere I wanted. Each district has its own department and the links with the local *dispensaire* are good. In theory at least the structure for community care works well here. Within each local department, there are wards for acute cases, for schizophrenics and for borderline cases. There is also a separate department of six geriatric wards, a research department and a forensic ward.

In the West, psychiatrists constantly complain of lack of funding. Dr Kosirev, the director of the Kashenko, explained that this wasn't really the problem. His hospital had money but he couldn't spend it on what he needed to buy. As we walked through one of the driveways, he pointed to the potholes. There were the roubles to mend the potholes. But, he shrugged, did I imagine it was possible to persuade the local controller of building services, the head of remontes, to provide labour to fill the holes? Never. Psychiatric hospitals weren't a priority. Now, to make matters worse, there was a building boom in Moscow. Perestroika and glasnost had made it possible for the papers to criticize the city's chronic housing shortage. All the labourers were at work on new apartment blocks or repairing old tenements, some of which dated back to the days of the Tsar. When we reached the ward we were walking to, Dr Kosirev pointed to a stack of marble slabs. He shrugged again. 'Actually, I've gone off the design,' he confided – but it had taken him months to get a date out of the local remonte for men to come to lay them.

The failure to maintain the fabric of the hospitals affects the treatment, Dr Kosirev said. It also meant that they rather despaired of solving the overcrowding problem.

It is hard to get precise statistics for the total hospital population of the USSR. The Soviet Union doesn't seem to give these to the World Health Organization. The only Eastern bloc countries that do so are Poland and Hungary. Dr Yastrebov, of the All Union Centre of Psychiatry, told me, however, that roughly 1 per cent of the country's population was schizophrenic. The population is 283 million which suggests 2.83 million are schizophrenic or have closely related disabilities. Yastrebov said that 17 per cent of these are in hospital. That would make for about 480,000 schizophrenic inpatients. The best statistics are for Moscow which has 16 psychiatric hospitals, 19 inpatient clinics and 7 psychosomatic wards in general hospitals. The city has about 23,000 beds, vastly more than London (Tichonenko 1988). It seems reasonable to suppose there are at least 600,000 inpatients. The lack of precise national statistics won't be surprising to anyone who knows the Soviet scene. The USSR has not published statistics in many areas because it wasn't considered proper, let alone necessary, to expose such state secrets. There are hardly, even now, any telephone directories and it's been admitted that many maps were deliberately falsified.

Patients, psychiatrists and even politicians agree there is gross overcrowding. Dr Potapov, the Minister of Health of the Russian Federation, told me there just hadn't been one new hospital built in the last five years from Moscow to the Pacific. I saw no single rooms in any hospital. Even in a privileged place like the Bechterev, a narrow room would have eight or ten beds. Patients didn't have cupboards and often not even a bedside table of their own.

Community care is yet to make any impact on the population of hospitals. The average stay of patients in hospital is quite long. The ordinary hospitals I visited said on average patients stayed between sixty and ninety days; in the UK, it's under 3 weeks.

The role, and rule, of the doctor

It will seem offensive to some Soviet psychiatrists to compare their practices with those of the Third World. I don't mean to be offensive, but some of their authoritarian attitudes to patients recall those of doctors in Egypt or India who have no doubt that they do what's best (Cohen 1988). No soft therapeutic manner consoles patients for the pain of depression or the miseries of schizophrenia. Later on in this chapter, I describe two interviews that were carried out by doctors who more or less barked at patients. This isn't just a bad bedside manner but betrays a generally patronizing, even contemptuous feeling. There was also a blatant disregard for privacy in the Kashenko.

This arrogance is perhaps even more remarkable because the Soviet Union uses some techniques which have been largely abandoned, like the magnetomachine in the *dispensaire*. In hospitals, insulin coma therapy and sleep therapy are routine. Soviet hospitals do not always find it easy to get the drugs they want. There isn't enough hard currency to buy them. Stellazine, widely used in the West as an anti-depressant, was no longer available. The Soviet Union does have a pharmaceutical industry of its own but a number of psychiatrists said there had been production problems. As we shall see in Chapter Ten, Western drug companies are waiting for what they expect to be a lucrative Soviet market to open. It would be wrong to suggest that patients always suffer from this lack of drugs. There are relatively few patients in ordinary hospitals who look over-medicated. Problems with drug supplies would seem, however, to keep some curious treatments very much in currency.

British hospitals are now run by committees. The post of medical superintendent has been abolished. But in the Soviet Union, hospitals have directors who are very influential. They clearly outrank other doctors and have privileges and status the rest can just dream of. In one hospital, the head of a number of departments complained bitterly that while his director often travelled to conferences abroad, he, who sweated it with the patients, had never been outside the USSR. The director has a large office with a large desk and, nearly always, either a portrait or a bust of Lenin. The glory of his office trumpets his power. Directors are usually appointed by Regional Departments of the Ministry of Health.

Dr Kosirev, the director of the Kashenko Hospital, who complained about the potholes, is a big man. He starts each day with a radio transmission from his office to the staff on all the wards. They report in to him with a list of the overnight problems and, from the centre, Kosirev radiates decisiveness and listens to his staff. Kosirev has been in charge of hospitals for some time. He used to be the director of Belgrade Hospital. He had been brought to the Kashenko clearly because there was concern about a scandal on the forensic ward. There, psychiatrists declared perfectly sane criminals to be insane – for a fee.

My dealings with Kosirev were the most normal of my dealings with any Soviet psychiatrist. When I first met him, he was intensely suspicious and rather curt. He wanted to know what I thought of the new law. Did I approve of it? He wouldn't really discuss anything till I'd put my cards on the table. I said that I thought it offered patients valuable protection, in theory at least.

Kosirev disagreed. The new law did have good points but it pained him. If he saw someone suffering, for example, if he passed someone who was having hallucinations on the street, his first instinct as a doctor was to help him. The new law would make that harder. But the fact that we disagreed didn't matter once I had convinced him I wasn't out to do a destructive job. Kosirev was willing to show more of himself than the other doctors. He spent part of one visit flirting with one of the production team and when, during another visit, I talked for a long time to one of his female psychologists, he teased, 'You're not being professional.' One of his hobbies is photography and he inquired earnestly about the cost of my Pentax. Getting some sense of his character was reassuring because most other psychiatrists remained very guarded. They would elaborate their positions on various aspects of medicine but remained hidden as people. Kosirev even eventually discussed at some length his involvement in one of the most celebrated of dissident cases, that of Grigorenko adding carefully he only saw him on his way out.

Admission routines

All new cases first go in through the admission procedure in a separate admissions building. Moscow has a special service of psychiatric ambulances which ferries in new patients. I observed a number of admissions, including that of a young soldier sent in by the army and an old lady of seventy-eight.

Maria had been sent to the Kashenko by an ordinary hospital. The hospital had been unable to find anything wrong with her. She arrived clutching her passport, a bag with an apple in it and some money. The ambulance men got her to sit down and the nurse signed her in. The nurse at once counted the money Maria had on her and shouted: 'That's 1 rouble and 56 kopecks. Got any more, Marischka?'

The admission room in which Maria sat was confusing. The phone was ringing constantly. In front of her, a doctor was busily scanning a computer screen. He wore a chef's hat and, of course, the regulation white coat. The chef's hat may have made him look exotic to me but, for Maria, that was normal dress for a doctor. He proceeded to conduct a very brisk clinical interview. He asked Maria her name and her date of birth. She said she had been born in 1910. He then asked her age. She said she was about forty. He then asked her what year it was.

'1937,' she said.

But if it was 1937 and she was born in 1910 she must really be twenty-seven. He had, I thought, a sly glint of triumph.

Maria didn't acknowledge his mathematics. She shrugged. Later, it turned out that one of her children had been born in 1937.

Her confusion had cause.

'What season is it?'

'Winter,' she said.

'What month is it?'

'January, I think.'

It was December and he repeated her answer. 'What date is it?' he demanded.

'I can't remember.'

'You can't remember, eh?' he said. 'Do you know where you are?'

'I'm in hospital.'

'But what kind of hospital?' he insisted.

'I don't know.'

There was no reason why she should know. It didn't look any different from any other hospital with its panoply of nurses wearing white hats. In the room next to the interview room, a room Maria had seen into, there was medical equipment. When she admitted that she didn't know what kind of hospital it was, the doctor didn't tell her.

'When did you start having problems with your memory?' he said.

'It got worse gradually,' Maria said.

'Ah, it got worse gradually,' he repeated. 'Is this the first time you have seen a psychiatrist?' he said, finally hinting where she was.

'Yes,' she said softly.

'You don't mind seeing a psychiatrist, do you?'

'No.'

The doctor was initially running through a standard set of questions for judging how confused elderly patients are. But he wasn't really listening to her. Maria wasn't completely confused. She was behaving quite appropriately in the strange situation she found herself in. She knew it was winter. She gave additional, and relevant information about her family. She had a son in the army and two daughters living in Moscow. She realized her memory was getting worse. There might well have been reasons to decide to keep her in hospital but they could have been discussed with her. Her memory wasn't so bad as to make her unable to decide anything for herself. The doctor didn't even tell her why he thought it necessary to admit her.

Under the new law of 1988 patients are supposed to be given the right to appeal against being brought into hospital. But Maria was never told this, let alone told that she, or her family, could contact a lawyer. The doctor didn't make inquiries about how else she might be cared for without entering the hospital. In about four minutes, he decided to admit her. I wasn't prepared for what happened next.

The nurse took off Maria's scarf and led her into the next room. Maria stood passively while the nurse undressed her. Then she was left standing naked in the middle of the room. The other hospital had sent her without any underwear. There didn't seem to be pressing reason to leave this old lady naked, as for the next few minutes all she did was wait. After a few minutes, Maria sat down and the nurse helped her off with her shoes. Then, again, nothing happened. A second nurse then asked Maria to walk over to the couch to have her blood pressure taken.

Maria didn't protest at any of this. Then she was taken to the next room which has a bath in the middle. There was no privacy. She had come in from another hospital so there was no reason to suppose she was dirty but she was washed in public. Broadmoor patients objected to such routines because they are fundamentally degrading (Cohen 1981). Maria was then taken to another room.

After about fifteen minutes, she was dressed and brought out to an ambulance. The grounds of the Kashenko are very large and she had to be driven to the geriatric ward.

Other admission patients were treated identically. The young soldier I saw was stripped by the nurses and also left waiting to have his blood pressure taken. He was, however, allowed to have a shower which was behind a curtain.

These procedures were not malicious, but the doctors in the admission department took them as perfectly routine. It was hard to watch them without concluding, however, that they did reflect a certain high-handed attitude. Patients weren't individuals so much as objects of medical intervention.

The main wards

Each district of Moscow has its own section of the Kashenko. On this section there are acute and chronic wards. The acute ward is locked, as are nearly all wards in all hospitals. The most remarkable thing as you enter is that most patients are wearing blue overalls. There is a hospital uniform which, rather unfairly, makes the place feel like a prison. Dr Kosirev said that they hoped to do something about the patients' clothes but it hadn't been possible yet. The staff were also in uniform. Nurses and doctors all wear radiant white and most also sport remarkable hats like the chef's hat the admission doctor wore. Clearly, no one must confuse the patients with the staff.

Most of the wards at the Kashenko have a very conventional design. Large bedrooms go off a long corridor. In the centre of the corridor, there is a dining area. Patients usually get their drugs here. As they were finishing breakfast, a nurse was walking round the tables giving out tablets. Near the entry door, there's a ward sitting room with jigsaw puzzles and a television set. Curiously, it is in this room that doctors interview patients.

The bedrooms are kept tidy and rather impersonal. In some rooms, there were bedside cabinets by each bed; in others, there weren't. Patients appeared to have very few possessions of their own. Dr Kosirev said that at times the wards did get overcrowded though things were better now than they had been before. In some bedrooms, there were five beds; in others up to twelve. The most overcrowded conditions I saw were in the geriatric ward with eleven patients crammed into one small room, all the beds touching each other.

At the Kashenko, patients are not allowed to be idle. On most wards they are responsible for cleaning their rooms. Noticeboards show what marks each room has been awarded for cleanliness. On the forensic ward, they went even further. A number of patients who were there to be assessed – were they responsible for their actions when they committed crimes? – were being paid to rebuild and redecorate a room. There was a large pile of bricks in the middle and they had just finished putting up a new rose-coloured wallpaper. The patients were glad to be working since it passed the time and meant that they could give money to their families. Given how hard it is for Soviet hospitals to arrange for building work to be done officially, this seems an interesting practice. I couldn't tell if pressure had been put on the patients to become navvies, but they didn't seem at all unhappy.

The male acute ward, rather drab and overcrowded, is typical of most of the Kashenko's wards. But in a few areas the hospital had clearly made an effort to create a pleasant environment. Dr Kosirev showed off a ward for geriatric neurotics that could have featured in *House and Garden*. Long-leaved plants had been carefully set up all over the sitting room; cheerful tapestries hung from the walls; the bedrooms had either two or four beds and looked cosy. Dr Kosirev was rightly proud of the ward. He stressed that it was the work mainly of the staff.

One of the paradoxes of Soviet psychiatry is that this practice of encouraging patients to work would seem to suggest an admirable measure of trust. If a man is intelligent enough to decorate a room, for instance, he ought to be intelligent enough to be involved in decisions concerning treatment. I was to witness this at its most dramatic as the psychiatrist in charge of the ward carried out her morning inspection of her patients.

As the doctor entered the ward sitting room, many patients were sitting down quite relaxedly. Flanked by two junior doctors, she went round from man to man. None got more than two or three minutes of her time. They were told to get up to talk to her. The first patient she talked to was a young boy with a crewcut who said he felt all right. She didn't accept this. She asked if he still had nightmares. He mumbled a maybe and then she told him that he looked ill. He should buck up his attitude.

Then it was the turn of a man who had been in the army. He looked like he was in his late thirties. His hair too was cut short. He stood stiffly to attention while she questioned him. The pose seemed right. First, she rebuked him for trying to boss other patients around 'because you're not in the army now'. Then she turned to his other deficiencies, especially abusing the fixtures and fittings.

The doctor demanded: 'Why did you kick the door out?'

'Where?' The patient shook his bemused head.

'In the toilet,' she insisted.

'I didn't.'

'But you did,' she repeated, 'you smashed it with your fist.'

'No.'

'No?' She then dropped the whole topic quite abruptly. 'You

weren't very nice to your wife when she came, and didn't talk to her. Why?'

He didn't answer at once and she moved a little closer to him. Finally, he mumbled, 'I don't know.'

She wasn't going to let him get away with that. 'Does she go out with other men like before?'

'Well, no. I'll sort it out.' He didn't want to talk about it, it seemed. That was hardly strange in the middle of the ward.

She had let all his fellow patients know that his wife was unfaithful but then didn't seem to finish the interview. Rather, she turned her attention to a younger man who was sitting down. He had a tattoo on his arm and looked quite tough. But he too rose to attention. He told her that he was frightened of children.

'What children?' she demanded.

He didn't at once reply.

'What children? What children terrorize you?'

'Some of those at school.'

'Your own or other people's?' she barked.

'I don't have any children of my own.'

She didn't seem pleased at having been corrected on that detail. 'Do all schoolchildren terrorize you?'

He repeated what he had said – that some children frightened him.

She carried on her rather intimidating round in much the same manner.

One explanation for this tough approach may well be that Soviet psychiatrists want to weed out malingerers who might be trying to avoid army service. Every Soviet boy spends three years in the army on national service. Pretending to be crazy has been a traditional way of getting out of it. In many cases when young men get to the army, they dislike the discipline and either genuinely become disturbed or feign madness. I talked to a number of middle-aged men who boasted of how their convincing craziness had allowed them to escape national service. In the Kashenko, I talked to one withdrawn young man who had a very reddened eye. He had just come to the hospital from the army. All he would say to explain being in hospital was 'it's an army problem'. But many of the men whom the doctor talked to abrasively were too old to be avoiding the army. She seemed just remarkably high-handed. Again, the patients weren't treated individually.

The patients

The patients in the acute ward were mainly schizophrenic. This was also true of patients in the Bechterev and at Kaluga. Soviet psychiatrists, as I argued in the chapter on the dissident controversy, tend to diagnose schizophrenia fairly widely. They also tend to strive for exceptionally precise diagnoses. Even though Vartanyan had said, wittily, that psychiatry wasn't a matter of mathematical equations, many of his colleagues would talk of the third or fourth order of psychosis. The Soviet journals carry remarkably convoluted diagnoses like 'A Clinico-Catamnestic Study of Patients with Episodic Progressive Schizophrenia exhibiting Affective, Anxious-Affective and Affective-Hallucinatory Episodes in childhood.' (Fall 1988. *Soviet Neurology*).

It is true that one could cull similar diagnostic follies out of the American DSM III, the standard US manual of psychiatric diseases. But, in practice, few Western psychiatrists believe you can dissect mental illnesses with quite such an exactitude. It shows how powerful the organic tradition still is that Soviet psychiatrists should use such unwieldy diagnoses. And this obsession to pin down the precise notch your paranoia has reached is even more curious because there is a very casual attitude to the kind of statistics Western doctors think useful. The Kashenko Hospital didn't have a breakdown of how many patients suffered from what category of illness but I was told that the main kinds of patients were schizophrenics, depressives, borderline states and geriatric cases. I had no reason to doubt that many Kashenko patients had classic symptoms of schizophrenia. One man told me that he had started hearing voices in his head and that his mother had sent him to the hospital. The acute ward also had a number of depressed patients. Boris had been an economist. His second marriage had broken up. He said he had been admitted in a very

miserable state three months before. He was now much better
thanks to a mixture of drugs and what the hospital calls 'psycho-
correction'.

Every time I visited the ward, it seemed to be rather quiet.
Most patients were just sitting around. A few played chess.
The wards in every hospital I visited carry timetables on their
noticeboard. In general, patients have to be up by 8 A.M.. They
finish breakfast by 9 A.M.. Then those who are able go to work.
At the Bechterev, some patients go to group therapy; at the
Kashenko, some go to play therapeutic games. But, in general,
Soviet patients are expected to spend the morning working.
Many hospitals take groups out to have a walk before lunch. I
was often told that walks were a traditional part of therapy.
Then, after lunch, most patients return to work though some
are allowed to have a nap. Few psychiatric hospitals the world
over are a hive of therapeutic activity. Soviet ones are no
exception. Time seems to hang heavy on the wards. People
often shuffle from one end of their ward to the other, or sleep.
An air of inactivity prevails. One interesting exception is the
ward on the Kashenko where they play therapy games which
are sometimes called 'psycho-correction'.

The use of such games in hospitals is relatively new in the
USSR apart from at the Bechterev Hospital. Dr Kosirev
explained that they had started these games at the Kashenko
about two years ago. Every morning, a group of patients –
some from the acute ward, some from the borderline wards –
spend two hours with psychologists. The group starts with an
exercise in mime. They all, including the staff, mimed their
way through washing their faces, brushing their teeth, shaving
and tying up their shoelaces. Many of the group smiled as they
went through the performance. Then Boris sat at one end of
the room with another patient by his side. In turn, every other
member of the group came up and asked, 'What will my fate
be?' Boris replied in sign language which the patient next to
him had to interpret. One 'dialogue' went:

'What will my fate be?'
Boris crossed his fingers.
'Prison,' explained his sidekick.

'I'm overjoyed,' replied the inquirer, laughing. The rest of the group laughed.

Later on, they played a game with blindfolds. Four patients sat at a table in the centre of the room and tried to draw a family while they were still wearing blindfolds. The rest of the group crowded in. Then they tried to draw a collective face. Both exercises provoked much laughter. It was the only time I heard laughter on any ward.

A student from Moscow University, Larisa, told me that she enjoyed the games 'because I see in them adaptation'. She had never done anything like it before but she thought it helpful 'because I am an optimist'. One of the few patients who didn't seem to be enjoying it all was the boy who had been rebuked in the ward for not owning up to his nightmares. Most of the patients who took part in these games came from the ward for borderline states. The theory was that they would build confidence and social skills.

After the schizophrenics, the next largest group of patients at the Kashenko are those suffering from depression. The same was true at the Bechterev and Kaluga. The reasons for their problems, and the circumstances that aggravated them, seemed familiar. People had become depressed when their marriages had broken down or when their loved ones had died. One woman had been ill ever since her son had died. 'I've never recovered from that,' she said, though it was twenty years ago. An old lady proudly showed off a scrapbook about her husband who had been in the army. They had been married forty-eight years when he died. His death had made her intensely depressed, 'though now I am coming out of it,' she smiled. She had a granddaughter living in Weybridge, Surrey, and hoped to visit her. The tales of unhappy lives were very similar to those one would find in the West.

However, there are some 'triggers' of depression that are distinctly Soviet. The most curious one is that life in the USSR is felt as such a psychological strain it provokes crises. People often complained that the hassles over getting food, dealing with bureaucracy and making sure one survived the slings and arrows of changing political orthodoxies caused vast stress. I can find no research evidence to back up this proposition but many Soviets believe it passionately. The West doesn't only have more consumer goodies but also more peace of mind, they feel. It's easier to catalogue more tangible sources of stress. Housing problems are so bad that often couples who divorce have to keep sharing the same accommodation, as Ludmilla was obliged to do. The Afghan war has taken its toll, as the Vietnam war did in America. There are many burnt-out soldiers in wards, though usually in army hospitals. Drink is a further complicating factor and there's been considerable debate in the Soviet literature about whether or not alcoholics should be treated in hospitals or in special facilities. There are some institutions where alcoholics are sent to dry out and work. In the Kashenko, I met a man on the borderline ward who was slightly manic. He laughed as he said that vodka had been his main drug, main joy, main problem. Before vodka took over his life, he had been a pilot for Aeroflot and then flew crop-spraying planes. He thought the hospital was 'marvellous'. His doctor took me aside and whispered, amused, 'He's very patriotic, you know, and you are a foreigner.'

An aesthetic approach

Many Soviet hospitals stress the value of 'aesthetic therapy'. The jargon shouldn't be allowed to over-impress. Aesthetic therapy means providing nice surroundings. In most psychiatric institutions that is difficult. At Kaluga Hospital, Dr Lifschitz, its director, proudly showed me round the women's neurotic ward. He had contacted a local artists' organization and had commissioned from them a series of murals for the ward. The murals of pretty country scenes inside and outside dominated the central part of the ward. They showed a family eating, animals in a farmyard and, even, a country church. Lifschitz's attitude isn't unique though he was quite willing to spend money on it.

At the Kashenko staff and patients provide the art. Apart from the plants in one women's ward, the forensic department specializes in sculpture. In the waiting room where inmates meet their families, there are gigantic wooden chairs, some in the shape of scallops; others in the shape of trees. Dr Kosirev pointed them out with pride. The main sitting room of the forensic ward also is highly decorated. 'I don't know why the patients drew this. The women aren't even naked,' Kosirev said provocatively.

Bringing in the Baptists to help

One of the consequences of the State's hostility to religion was that it stopped nearly all voluntary work. Groups of young Communists did sometimes provide additional help on wards but this was rare. Generally, everything in hospitals had to be done by the staff.

Perestroika has had an interesting effect here. As the State's attitude to religion has softened, enterprising hospital directors have brought in both Orthodox and Baptist groups to provide a variety of useful services. According to Godfrey Hoskins in the 1988 Reith lectures, the Orthodox Church traditionally prided itself on its sense of community. Its faith shone through its pastoral work. But decades of co-operating with the State in order to survive robbed the Orthodox Church of spiritual energy. The Baptists have taken advantage of this opportunity, Hoskins suggests, and have become one of the most successful Churches in the Soviet Union. They're now also providing much-needed help for nothing.

The geriatric ward at the Kashenko is grim. It has some of the most overcrowded rooms in the hospital. There is less to do than in other wards. In one room old ladies roll together white bits of string. Their faces look sad and, throughout the ward, there's a sour stench. There seemed to be far less staff here than on the other wards.

'I'd pay the people on the geriatric ward most if I could,' Kosirev said. Their work is the most demanding. Oddly, given his concern, the geriatric ward seemed to have the fewest staff. The relaxation of attitudes to religion meant that it was possible for Kosirev to bring in some Baptists to provide assistance the staff needed badly.

Tanya Zarik is one of six Baptists who work regularly on the geriatric ward. She has a family and a job so she explained she could only come one day a week. Tanya is in her thirties and very fresh-looking. She was dressed like a member of staff in a white coat though she didn't have the nurse's hat. Instead she wore a scarf. Tanya explained that the volunteers did things the nurses didn't have time to do. They talked to the patients, fed those who couldn't feed themselves, read to them, tried to cheer them up. Tanya liked reading them poems. Her fellow Baptist, Vera, was brushing an old woman's hair and discussing what she liked to eat.

The spirit of perestroika was very much in evidence in all this. Tanya said, 'We don't meet any problems. The staff give us their support.' She emphasized that they were not muzzled. 'No one harasses us. We can talk about God and our faith.' I imagined that she talked a good deal about her faith, for she was something of an evangelist and invited us all to come to a huge Sunday service.

'The Baptists have become friends,' said one lady. Others agreed.

Yet, again, there are limits. There are no religious services available at the Kashenko. I also found it hard to get to the bottom of just how the Baptists had started to work on the ward. Dr Kosirev was not very specific. He just said that it had seemed a good idea and there had been no problem implementing it. He pointed to an article in the *New York Times* which reported on the first days of the Baptist experiment. But that article wasn't clear either on how it had all started. Yet, like the therapy games, the involvement of religious groups is a sign of positive change.

The Kashenko may, however, be exceptional. Neither at the Bechterev nor in Kaluga did anyone mention such voluntary workers.

The forensic ward

One sign of the close link between care and control is that many hospitals have forensic wards where patients on criminal charges are sent to be assessed. The ordinary hospital in Tallin has such a department, as does the Kashenko. In Chapter Three, I reported on the scandal at the Kashenko's forensic ward where criminals had paid lavishly to get a diagnosis.

The Kashenko ward is large. It houses up to sixty patients. Each of the bedrooms has about ten beds and some beds are packed along a corridor. All the patients wear blue uniforms. They spend a month or two in the ward. In theory these are the most dangerous patients in the hospital. The ward is locked and there's a visiting room which is also locked. The windows are all barred. Dr Kosirev explained that they wanted to remove the bars but they had been so solidly set into the bricks it was proving impossible. The patients might be there to be assessed but they were also there to work. Dr Kosirev showed off the small swimming pool they had built in the forensic garden.

On a Sunday, the visiting room was like a busy railway terminal. The room was packed with families. There was food all over the place as many visitors had brought hot meals for their relatives. One old lady was feeding her son, who must have been thirty, beef stew from a saucepan. Another woman was handing her son tea and cakes. The little groups were intense and noisy.

Since the scandal, the patients who were sent for assessment to the Kashenko are those who have committed less serious crimes like assault, minor robbery and domestic offences. A psychologist who wore a very stylish white dress said 'I don't wear the hospital uniform for the staff. It creates barriers.' Her role was to help the psychiatrists reach a decision about whether or not the man was responsible for his actions.

I sat in while she interviewed Viktor who had attacked his wife's lover. 'He does not want us to find him not responsible,' she explained, 'because there is the custody of the child at stake. He wants the child.' If the hospital judged him too ill to answer the case, he would have little hope of getting his child.

She asked Viktor how he felt and then started to give him a colour test. He had to choose which of a number of colours he liked and which he disliked. As a result of his choices, she was sure she could tell how responsible he was.

The care Soviet patients receive in ordinary hospitals has been criticized both by ex-patients and by politicians like Potapov. It's hardly strange that many of the poor practices ordinary patients suffered from should also affect the 'politicals'.

6

Serbsky

'The Serbsky is like a hotel,' said Podrabinek, 'but it's a hotel on the way to hell.' Once a 'political' was sent to the Serbsky, his fate was sealed. Years in a special hospital lay ahead, Podrabinek said.

No one knows for sure how many dissidents came to the Serbsky to be diagnosed. Grigorenko, Bukovsky, Medvedev and Plyusch were perhaps the most famous to be assessed by its staff. The West saw the Serbsky as the central cog of the whole system. Bloch put it succinctly: 'The Serbsky was the apex of the abuse'. In this chapter, I want to describe what the Serbsky is like now, to report on who its current patients are and to attempt to see whether it is still dealing with dissidents.

The Soviets see the Serbsky as a very necessary part of their criminal justice system. Its job is to assess any person charged with a crime who may not be responsible for his actions. Under Soviet law, a defendant may ask to be examined. Often, defendants do claim to be mentally ill. But the prosecution can argue, or the court itself can rule, that a defendant is not able to defend himself. The harshest critics accept that most of those the Serbsky saw committed ordinary non-political crimes. But Bloch and Reddaway argued that one whole ward, Ward 4, with thirty-four beds in it, was specifically designed for political cases. 'All the tricky political cases came here,' Bloch said. The best way to avoid embarrassing cases in open court was to send someone to be assessed at the Serbsky. Its psychiatrists were always eager to oblige and use their 'expertise' to spare the State trouble.

Though psychiatrists tend to be wary of criticizing colleagues, many have been acid about the Serbsky and its director Georgy

Morosov. Bloch has accused him of 'numerous half truths' and possibly some outright lies. John Wing of the Maudsley has also been cutting about the way Dr Morosov has handled controversies, accusing him of writing untruths to the *British Medical Journal*. On the Soviet side, there is also anger. The Serbsky staff argue they are doing a difficult job in difficult circumstances. Accusations about their honesty can only be due to cold war stereotypes and the lust of the Western press for a sensational tale of Bolshevik evil. It's against this background of accusation and counter-accusation that I try to describe the Institute.

The Serbsky was founded in 1921 by Vladimir Serbsky, who had been head of the Rimsky Korsakov Institute. Serbsky had crossed swords with the Tsar's government in 1911, for he claimed that many of the psychiatric illnesses Russians suffered from were due to poor social conditions. An unjust society took its toll. Serbsky's Institute is called the Institute of Forensic and General Psychiatry. He never intended it to be devoted exclusively to criminal work.

The forensic work of the Serbsky involves two difficult areas: assessing how responsible a person was for a crime and predicting how dangerous they are likely to be. How dangerous a person is reckoned to be will influence both what kind of hospital they go to and when they can be released. Assessing responsibility and dangerousness aren't easy skills in any society (Rack 1982). The perfect patient, not too deferential, may just have learned how to play the rules of the therapeutic games, just to fool the psychiatrists. Outside, in the real world, in a crisis, he kills again.

The main Serbsky buildings are a drab complex in Kropotokin Street in central Moscow. There's a peculiar irony to this location, for Prince Kropotokin was a famous Victorian anarchist who was always in trouble with the Tsar. He was often imprisoned and, had he been alive in Communist times, he might well have found himself being assessed in the Serbsky.

The entrance hall is dim. You give your name, your reason for visiting and the person expecting you to a receptionist who sits behind a grille. She was fairly fearsome even though I and our Soviet colleagues were expected. Usually, you have to wait before you can proceed further. In the entrance hall, notices say how much bread, sugar and other 'luxuries' relatives can bring to inmates. Children under sixteen are not allowed to visit.

The entrance procedure is both grim and comic. At one end of the entrance hall there's a strong wooden door. When it's your turn, you are told to press a buzzer. The militia inside look at you and then press a corresponding buzzer to open the door. You walk into an extremely narrow space like an airlock. The next door will not open till the one behind it has been closed. The first time I went through, a woman who glanced up menacingly at me, nodded and then resumed a row she was having with the receptionist. The inquisitorial gaze of authority is a look perfected by the Soviet militia. At Moscow airport, they even have a mirror set up behind passengers so that the militia can look you up, down and behind. The relentless scrutiny is grim but what seems comic is that nearly all the security equipment is antiquated. The doors creak. The locks are old. In theory, the two doors should never be held open at the same time but often they're both held open. In three visits, I never saw anyone searched.

Inside the buildings are grouped around a courtyard. Nearly all the walls are dirty white. In some parts derelict equipment lies about. On one wall, there is a camera surveying the grounds. Some windows have bars: others have been white-washed so that you can't see in or out. At the bottom of the building that houses Ward 3, the only ward I was allowed to visit, there were four militia men but they weren't exactly on alert guard. They were lounging around puffing at cigarettes. Again, the security seems baffling. It is supposed to be tight yet at the back of part of the yard boxes are stacked against the wall so an agile patient could leap over to freedom.

On my first visit, I was taken into a building with many blacked-out windows. Wire mesh ran alongside the staircase 'to prevent patients throwing themselves over and committing suicide,' Dr Miluhin said. He is head of the international department and, in Dr Morosov's absence, was one of four senior psychiatrists I met. They had rather different views about whether they would give permission for filming. Miluhin attacked the way the Serbsky had been pilloried in the press and made a spirited defence of sluggish schizophrenia. He laughed a shade aggressively, 'Wouldn't it be nice, though, if we could show you a sluggish schizophrenic. That would make your programme a hit.' Yet Miluhin seemed to take it for granted the film would happen. The second doctor remained entirely silent throughout.

The other two, Shostakovitch and Alexandrovsky (of Transmash), were less hostile yet more uncertain about filming. They said sluggish schizophrenia was only rarely used as a diagnosis and then in examinations only. They made the point that the USSR still had the death penalty. If they decided that a man who had been convicted of murder or corruption was insane, it would save his life.

I ended that first meeting rather sceptical about their assurance that they were keen to see the film made, especially as I wasn't allowed to set foot on any of the wards.

My next two visits, however, gave me a clearer picture. There are six wards. Two are for schizophrenic cases, one is for borderline patients. One is a women's ward. One deals with civic cases and there is a children's ward. I was told the Serbsky houses between 230 and 250 patients at any one time.

There is also a psychology department though it is very subservient to the doctors. The first day I visited Ward 3, it was very overcrowded. Forty-three patients shared three rooms. The beds were crowded together. The corridors a dingy green and echo. The locks, like everything else, are very rickety. Nearly all the patients wore blue overalls though one man sported a brown leather jacket and another one floral pyjamas. He also had sunglasses which contrived to make him look like a banana republic dictator whose coup had misfired. Shostakovitch did not allow me to talk to the patients in case 'it agitates them'. It was an exceptionally rapid tour.

Outside the ward building is an exercise yard. The ward timetable in Ward 3 states that patients can spend two hours in the afternoon doing sports. I wasn't shown any sports facilities so perhaps this means they walk round the yard.

It was only on my second visit that I met Dr Morosov, the director of the Serbsky. He is an elegant-looking man with a splendid turf of grey hair. He has four gold teeth which give him a slightly sinister appearance. In the USSR gold teeth are fashionable, however.

Dr Morosov's suite of rooms at the Serbsky is palatial. There's a fine portrait of Serbsky and above Dr Morosov's head hangs a portrait of Lenin. Morosov's desk is plush as are the black leather armchairs dotted round the room. In no other medical institution was there this luxury. Only here were we served black caviar. I don't mean to sound churlish but the lavishness seemed excessive. Other doctors and professionals were crammed into small, rather cramped spaces. The opulence in Morosov's office was offputting given the poverty of the wards.

Dr Morosov is a fluent talker and when I asked him to explain the work of his Institute, he spoke non-stop for ten minutes. Every time I tried to put a question, he steam-rollered his way through it. Often he repeated himself. The actual amount of information he gave was relatively small and, again, surprisingly imprecise. He said the majority of inmates had committed rape, assaults, hooliganism and theft of state and of private property. He did not mention murders or debt. Apart from the 250 patients inside, others who were trusted were being assessed on an outpatient basis.

Dr Morosov agreed they were still assessing people who had been charged with political offences under article 190 of Soviet legislation. 'There was a period when there were more such people but today the percentage has been considerably reduced.' He then waxed lyrical about the new freedoms. Under glasnost, 'You know now people can say what they want in our country and it isn't a crime.' Only those who were aggressive as well as outspoken now got into trouble with the law.

The Serbsky didn't have the right to refuse to assess a patient. 'That isn't our competence.' He repeated a number of times that their expertise was psychiatric assessment. It's important to be fair on this point. Some Western critics wrote as if psychiatrists could refuse to assess those on particular charges. The heroic course of action would have been to challenge the KGB and ask why it should be an offence to criticize. Psychiatrists in every country, however, administer the existing law apart from a few committed radicals. The only realistic case the West has against the Serbsky is that it didn't exercise its professional judgment properly.

When the courts send a patient to the Serbsky, the Institute appoints a commission of psychiatrists to examine him. The commission interviews him. Dr Shostakovitch said that their main method of working was through clinical interviews (which I was not allowed to sit through). Nearly all the patients also go through a routine of psychological tests. The director of the psychology department, Dr Kudyaseyev, let me see two of these tests in action. Earnest psychologists were getting patients to re-create a particular pattern using building blocks; in another room, they were getting a patient to sort some rather old cards into categories. Did the patient twig that a car, a plane and a boat should all be stacked together as forms of transport? Such tests are fundamentally IQ tests. They may reveal if a patient has abnormally low intelligence but not much else. The psychologists also use imprecise tests of motivation like Rorschach tests (where the patient says what an inkblot reminds him of) and TAT pictures (where he has to make up a story based on the picture and the story allegedly reveals the deeper motivation). Rather pathetically, Dr Kudyaseyev assured me that they only used tests which the West had approved of. I wasn't to think, he seemed to be saying, that they were using unreliable Soviet tests. Everything was of international standard. The whole process of interviewing and testing is supposed to take a month, but sometimes it takes longer. The Institute then tells the courts it needs more time.

The Serbsky's commission present their findings to the court. Dissidents did sometimes try to call other psychiatrists on their behalf as Kudyaseyev did. But, usually, the courts have taken the line that the expertise on offer at the Serbsky is the best available. Challenges were not welcome.

Dr Morosov explained that the Serbsky took referrals from all over the USSR. Whenever a local forensic facility couldn't cope, it sent patients to the Institute. The psychiatric literature acknowledges that the two areas the Serbsky deals in are rather nebulous in free societies. There are no clear symptoms which decree if a person is or is not responsible for his actions. A person could be very depressed and yet know quite well what he was doing when murdering his wife. Decisions about how dangerous patients can be are no easier. It seems that psychiatrists predict correctly how dangerous a patient will be on about 30 per cent of occasions. This is better than chance but far from perfect. These are complex judgments.

In the Soviet Union, the issues surrounding offences involving dissent made such clinical judgments even more complex. Assume for a moment that the psychiatrist was ethical and sensible. As a sensible person in the days before perestroika, our hypothetical psychiatrist would know that the Soviet Union was a totalitarian state. The Soviet Constitution did offer citizens many freedoms in theory but, in practice, bureaucracy ruled. To attempt to assert democratic rights in such a state could be seen as heroic, aggressively asking for trouble, or confused and rather strange. It is easy to see how psychiatrists could slip from seeing such behaviour as rather strange to seeing it as sick – especially given their attitude to ordinary patients. I am not seeking to condone the Serbsky but it is important to understand, as Segal tried to, how 'dissident' activity would have looked from the inside.

The view of critics has been much harsher. Bloch and Reddaway rely on Nekipelov, a poet who described the Serbsky in *The Institute of Fools* (1974). They say he 'discussed with imagination and compassion the formative influences on these doctors pointing to the ironic fact that while part of their time went on proving sane dissenters insane against their will, most of the rest went on frustrating the will of criminals who were simulating mental illness to try to avoid fifteen-year terms in camps or the death penalty'. Nekipelov concludes that the doctors were consciously unethical. 'Their motives are mostly the humdrum ones of careerism and intellectual and political conformism, vices often laced with straightforward cynicism, laziness or stupidity.' Later in the book, Bloch and Reddaway return to the question of psychiatrists' motives and argue that most Soviet psychiatrists never believed in sluggish schizophrenia or the insanity of dissidents. Bloch and Reddaway seem to believe that patients can not be abused if doctors sincerely believe their treatment is correct.

But there's considerable evidence that doctors sometimes abase patients though their intentions were good. (Gostin 1977: Cohen 1988).

With Dr Morosov's approval, my second visit to Ward 3 was more leisurely. The number of patients was down to thirty-five. The sad, tense atmosphere on the ward became obvious. Patients spend much of their day waiting for psychiatrists to talk to them. Meanwhile, the nurses watch them. It's not easy to be normal in any hospital. The overcrowding and the lack of exercise space make it hard. Men sat on their beds, or wandered restlessly. I saw few books. Through the tannoy a horrid tinny Muzak played. The Serbsky has not been accused of treating inmates badly during their short stay as Alexander Podrabinek joked sadly.

But the most surprising thing was the way in which patients were ready to talk. The doctors urged me to talk to one man who wore floral pyjamas. He was the most flattering about the Institute. The other three patients I interviewed offered themselves.

Nikolai, a dramatic-looking, thin man who fiddled constantly with his beard, had spent ten years in special hospital and wouldn't tell me what for. At first he seemed lucid. He said it was paradise here by comparison. But then he began to talk excitedly about his project, constructing the equation for human happiness. He scribbled furiously and gave me a copy of his equation.

The other patients seemed far less disturbed.

Mikhail was a small soft-spoken man. He asked to be interviewed. He sat down on his bed and outlined what life had been like in Oryol special hospital where he had spent three-and-a-half years. 'Everything that patients have is literally taken away from them, from the food in the canteen to the welding apparatus which was stolen recently. Working in special hospitals is a good fiddle for those who are there.' The discipline he had experienced was very strict. 'Let me only say that going to the toilet was a problem because you could only go at the times they decreed. The place was also very dirty with lice, parasites.'

Special hospitals do let patients read newspapers and Mikhail had learned that they had been transferred to the Ministry of Health from 1 April 1988. 'But it seems to have made practically no difference. There are the same watch towers and the same machine guns.' He hoped he would now be freed.

The patient who had been volunteered praised the Serbsky, but it was the fourth man, Ivan, who was the most interesting. He was a walking encyclopaedia of the Soviet health care system, after spells in Krasnodar, Chernyakhovsk and other hospitals. All the ward staff listened as he said:

'I was in Krasnodar. They put four people in two beds there, four people in two beds. Or people had to sleep on the floor. It was very dirty and the male nurses treated you not as human beings but like animals. That kind of treatment was very upsetting.'

He found treatment at the Serbsky was better. 'Here, they treat you with care and warmth. Not like a dog.' They had 'kultur', were civilized. It's true, of course, that the one institution he didn't criticize was the institution he was in.

He confirmed Mikhail's criticisms of the special hospital system for he had been the victim of theft. 'It happens too that nurses steal something from your food parcel. Then if you complain, you're given injections. To punish you for being truthful.' It had happened to him at Chernyakhovsk.

There wasn't, as there had been with Ephraim, a major attempt to discredit all this evidence. Dr Shostakovitch did reveal some details about their cases but conceded there were 'good special hospitals and some bad one'.

Dr Shostakovitch added that he now had no article 190 cases (political cases) on the wards. That might have been so, but the story that Ivan gave of how he had been admitted suggests that it is still not a good idea to cross the authorities.

Ivan said that after he had been in hospital, he returned to Donetsk to find that he had lost his flat. He went to the chairman of the local Soviet in his district to complain and ask for his flat back. 'I had no money so I asked him. Did you have breakfast today? Yes. Did you have lunch? Yes. Are you going to have dinner? Yes. I added that I just wanted to have those things too.' The chairman, Ivan alleged, said that they would do something for him. Then he was told to go away. As he said this story, Ivan's tone was very soft and Yelena said later that he spoke in a very nice way. I asked him if he had offered any violence. 'No,' he said, 'that wasn't in my character.'

Shostakovitch confirmed this and revealed the curious fact that a number of patients were in the Serbsky because of long-standing debt. I tried without success to clarify this. Three of the patients on the ward were in debt.

Despite the many criticisms that patients made, there was none of the panic of the *dispensaire*. The only sign of that emerged after we had left the ward. Dr Miluhin suddenly insisted that we only show the patients in silhouette, a condition that had never been mentioned before. Then Dr Morosov's assistant said that the doctors were very worried they would get into trouble because they had broken the law. He made this dramatic pronouncement as we were packing the gear to leave. The patients were under the protection of the court, he explained. Information about them was confidential. It wasn't clear whether the psychiatrists felt that they might be repri-manded because they let patients talk at all or because they allowed them to be identified or because they had given us some confidential information to set their cases in context.

No one seemed to know what to do. I decided to remain affable and vague. No one was asking for my tapes so I hoped it would reassure them if I said that I didn't want to do anything to get the doctors in trouble. Miraculously that seemed to be enough.

The Serbsky is well aware of its bad reputation outside the USSR. Dr Shostakovitch said that in most forensic departments around the USSR only about 10 to 15 per cent of cases were found to be mentally ill. As the most difficult cases came to the Serbsky their tally is higher, about 30 per cent. Among dissi-dents, however, the percentage declared mad is much higher, according to Bloch.

In the last twenty-five years, according to Western sources, perhaps 50,000 people charged either with anti-Soviet activities or attempting to cross the border have passed through the

Serbsky. In addition, a number of dissidents have been accused of ordinary crimes involving violence. The Serbsky deny that there was, or is, a special department for political cases. I certainly did not see one but my access was restricted. The wards were classified according to diagnostic categories.

Dr Morosov, one of the key advocates of sluggish schizophrenia, was often forceful when we talked but he never took the hostile tone of the letter to the WPA in 1983. He did not deny that there had been mistakes. 'We have made mistakes but when we make them, we acknowledge them.' He denounced the view, though, that there had ever been mistakes made for political reasons or that, 'Owing to political reasons, we had declared a healthy person mentally ill. That is an outright lie.'

The staff at the Serbsky, Morosov suggested, were themselves victims of abuse and Western deceit. American and European psychiatrists had come to see him, they had been allowed to roam the Institute and had assured him they were impressed. Back home, it was a different story. They published highly critical pieces.

There have been, however, a number of well-documented cases in which Western psychiatrists have complained of the way the Serbsky reported their visits.

John Wing, an eminent British psychiatrist, made a visit to the Serbsky in 1972. Wing had been on a general tour and had certainly found some Soviet services good, especially those for the chronically handicapped. The following report of the Serbsky visit appeared in the *Korsakov Journal*:

In the course of a day thirteen foreign psychiatrists were informed in detail about the position of forensic psychiatry in the Soviet Union, they took part in the examination of a patient and they familiarized themselves with the case histories of those patients whose names are used in the foreign press for slanderous anti-Soviet propaganda. Two foreign psychiatrists who expressed the desire to do visited one of these patients right in his hospital.

After the end of this session the foreign psychiatrists who had taken part in it made a favourable judgment about the professional level and the methods of psychiatric diagnosis of the Institute of Forensic Psychiatry named after V. P. Serbsky.

Wing countered: 'This is characteristic of the way the meeting has been reported in the Soviet Press in spite of my own statements to the contrary both to the Press and to the *British Medical Journal*.' Wing and the other Western forensic psychiatrists had been critical of Soviet practice. Dr Alfred Freedman, then the director of the American Psychiatric Association, explained why to the *New York Times* (1973). But Morosov reiterated that this group has all agreed that the 'five so-called dissidents they saw were rightly diagnosed irresponsible'.

Wing replied again to the *BMJ* that this was just not true. 'I have no doubt that many of my colleagues were not satisfied as I myself was not, that all five political dissenters whose cases we heard were so seriously mentally ill during the time of their legal examination as to be unfit to plead, to conduct their own defence or to instruct defence lawyers.'

In 1988, Morosov told Erik Seisby, a Danish professor and a member of the International Helsinki Federation, that a number of foreign psychiatrists had praised the Serbsky's work after seeing it. He referred in particular to a John Wing. It was remarkable that Morosov should do so. Wing was still bitter enough to make a statement to the International Association Against the Political Abuse of Psychiatry after the Seisby meeting.

The Wing incident was not the only one. Finn Magnussen, clinical director of the Ungdomspsykiatrisk Klinik in Norway, had visited the Serbsky in 1982 with three other Norwegian psychiatrists to explain why the Norwegian Pyschiatric Association would vote for the exclusion of the Soviets from the WPA. They hoped also to explore how 'a transcultural perspective on psychiatry might help understand our differences'. The Norwegian delegation didn't come prepared to see patients. It didn't, for example, have its own interpreter.

In 1988, Magnussen found that Morosov had told the International Helsinki Federation delegation a different story. Morosov said that the group had been invited to interview patients but had refused. This refusal wasn't innocent. Morosov added that, 'Magnussen had allegedly admitted that he had refused to examine the patient in question because he knew in reality the patient was sick.' Magnussen denies the charge as a 'complete fabrication'. But, Morosov would find it useful to suggest that Western psychiatrists couldn't face interviewing truly sick dissidents.

Morosov's attacks on the dishonesty of Western psychiatrists lack conviction. He was equally acerbic, however, about what happened to dissidents who left. He asked Western psychiatrists to publish details about cases of émigrés who lapsed back into mental illness after they left the USSR. He had had extensive correspondence with Austrian psychiatrists about an ex-patient called Christian but the Austrians refused to do the decent thing. Dr Morosov presented himself as more sinned against than sinning even though, of course, he was asking colleagues to release confidential information on patients.

The burden of evidence that the Serbsky diagnosed people inappropriately remains considerable. The conditions inside the Institute aren't savage but they certainly aren't good. Moreover, the fact that the Serbsky doesn't have so many political cases now is the result not of any change in psychiatric practice but in legal attitudes. Dr Morosov was accurate in saying that it is now, as of late 1988, possible to express all manner of views freely. Many of the political activities that were seen as criminal are now seen as a necessary part of the process of democratization. The conditions no longer create dissidents for the Serbsky to assess.

Ironically, given the West's view of the Serbsky, inside the Soviet Union it's seen as a miracle of honesty. It perhaps isn't surprising that Dr Vartanyan should mention that when Medvedev was detained at Kaluga Hospital, it was Serbsky psychiatrists who said this had been a mistake, a generous assessment of their role. Critical journalists like Andrei Mann of the *Medical Gazette* have been impressed also. Mann told me that when there were allegations of corruption at the Kashenko, the Serbsky was asked to examine patients. Mann concluded that the Serbsky psychiatrists acted quite properly.

Morosov is no longer president of the USSR Association of Psychiatrists but this move doesn't seem to have been made as a concession to Western pressure, for Dr Morosov is now an honorary President of the Association. His elevation is a sign of the failure of Soviet psychiatry to listen to some criticisms.

7

The Special Hospital System

The special hospitals were, for Western critics, the most horrifying aspect of the Soviet psychiatric system. Bloch and Reddaway called the American edition of their 1984 book, *Psychiatric Terror*. Dr Bloch explained to me that he felt it was a perfectly justified title especially given conditions in special hospitals. It's important, however, not to look at the Soviet special hospitals as if there were nothing else so awful in the rest of the world. Many Western countries have special hospitals for the criminally insane. Usually, inmates are sent to them because they are thought too dangerous for ordinary hospitals. Soviet psychiatrists justify sending patients to special hospitals on identical grounds. The special hospitals of democratic countries haven't been sweet institutions. Britain has seen well-documented scandals in Broadmoor and Rampton. MIND has just demanded an inquiry after the death of a Broadmoor patient in a cell. In the USA and in Norway, there have been scandals involving allegations of brutality in similar institutions. In this chapter, I report on what one special hospital is like and try to assess the whole system.

For Sergei Belov, it was a surprise to be sent to Volgograd Special Hospital. He was in an ordinary psychiatric hospital when, one morning, he was told to get dressed. He asked the sister why. She told him he was going somewhere else. Once he was dressed, he was handcuffed and told he was going to a special hospital. He was to spend three-and-a-half years in there, three-and-a-half years that have left him very angry.

The Soviet Union has at least sixteen special hospitals. During the period we were filming, responsibility for them was transferred from the Ministry of the Interior and the KGB to the Ministry of Health. There is some controversy as to the dates of the actual transfer.

Dr Stashkin, the director of the Leningrad Special Hospital, said that to some extent Western pressure led to the transfer. It didn't look good if the Ministry of the Interior, which had links with the KGB, had authority over the hospital. Being under the Ministry of Health would present a softer image. But the transfer was not going smoothly. There were rows about budgets between the different Ministries. Dr Potapov, the Minister of Health in the Russian Federation, told me that two of the special hospitals were in such a bad condition that his Ministry refused to accept them from the Interior. I pressed him to name these two but he refused to do so. He was keener to insist that they would not be accepted till their condition had been improved.

Many of the special hospitals are in the wilds; in Alma Ata on the Mongolian border, in Tashkent in central Asia, in Oryol, in Volgograd, in Chernyakhovsk, in Dnepropetrovsk in the Ukraine, and in Kazan, a hospital for women. In general the principle seems to be to locate these institutions as far away from Moscow as possible. Officially I was told that patients were sent to the special hospital that was closest to their family to make visiting easy, but I found little evidence of such consideration on the part of the authorities. Putting hospitals far from Moscow had an extra advantage. It made it hard for information about them to filter out.

As a result, the West has relied on information from a few sources like the Working Group in the seventies and, now, the continuing work of a few brave human rights monitors like Alexander Podrabinek. But few Western psychiatrists and no Western journalists had been allowed to visit the special hospitals. Of all the taboo institutions they were the most taboo. It wasn't surprising that most of them should be isolated.

The Leningrad Special Hospital is the exception. It is not isolated. It is at no 9 Arsenalya, a road that goes down to the Neva river. The hospital is five minutes' drive from the centre of the city. Opposite is a factory. This little patch of Leningrad also houses a women's prison which broods over the river. The special hospital itself was itself originally a prison. It looks very much like a grim Victorian institution. The buildings are mainly grey brick and, by now, rather grimy. Some of the walls are topped with strands of barbed wire.

You enter the hospital through a small, grim door that gives on to the road. Inside is a dark entrance hall. Unlike the Serbsky, there are no notices here telling relatives what they could bring.

At the entrance, you meet the stamp of its security. In all the secure Soviet institutions, the security looks rather antiquated. Entrance to the hospital is controlled by the militia men who stand in a booth behind bars. At the Serbsky, the operation of this system was casual. Here it was rigorous, even though we were expected.

You enter through a barred door into a courtyard. Barbed wire guards the wall on either side. The next building through the courtyard is the administrative building. The hospital director, Dr Stashkin, complained endlessly of the old buildings. He's had a wall in the administrative building painted a flashy shade of green. This bright wall stands out as a desperate attempt to inject gaiety. To get to the wards, you have to pass through another set of security gates. Militia men control the way in, and the way out, through another heavy door.

The hospital used to house Bukovsky and Fainberg. In his account of it, Bukovsky (1978) noted that there were armed guards as well as detention cells. One day, he tried to help a patient who was being attacked by the staff and he 'was punched so hard that I was sent flying under the bed and barely able to crawl out again.' (p. 161). Bukovsky complained of beatings, the fear of indefinite confinement and the irony that you couldn't complain 'for every complaint got lodged in your case register as yet one more proof of insanity.'

My account is not exhaustive as I wasn't given total access in the Leningrad Hospital. I got to see one rehabilitation ward, the medical treatment ward, some of the workshops and, by accident, an intensive treatment ward. The other evidence on the special hospitals I have comes from talking mainly to ex-patients like those at the Serbsky.

Dr Stashkin has been working at the hospital since 1975 and in charge of it since 1983. He is a clean-cut good looking man who was a little nervous at our visit. No journalists had been inside the special hospital and in the summer of 1988, a few months before we visited, there had been a group of psychiatrists including Dr Beyaert from Holland. 11 June, 1988 N. R. C. Handelsblad Beyaert wrote a very acid piece in which he mused on how the staff prevented riots as the security on the wards seemed relaxed. Were drugs being fed into the atmosphere? Given the reputation of the special hospitals, I could understand his sense of being baffled. It's a sign of the paranoia you can begin to feel that I wondered why I smelt a very strong odour of salami. Was there a salami-scented tranquillizer which tamed the patients? Did the doctors have gas masks to put on the moment inquisitive visitors from the West had gone?

Dr Stashkin explained that the majority of those in his hospital had committed murder; 40 to 45 per cent was the figure he gave. The rest were rapists, robbers, hooligans and had attempted murder. A very small number, perhaps 1 per cent, had committed minor acts like theft. He agreed that there had been in the past a number of patients who had been convicted under article 190 and of other political charges but there had never been many such patients. At most, he suggested they had made up 1 per cent of the hospital's population.

'There are no such patients now,' he said.

The average length of stay in the hospital was three-and-a-half years. There were patients who were there for as little as six months but, on the other hand, one man had been there for twenty-three years. He had murdered seven times and raped eight women in the space of a week. They were his enemies, he explained, because they had blue eyes.

The hospital had two admission wards, three treatment wards, two wards for very aggressive patients, three rehabilitation wards, one clinical ward and a medical ward. On all of them, Dr Stashkin said, they used conventional forms of treatment – drugs, some ECT, some forms of psychotherapy. He claimed they tried to get families involved in treatment.

Bloch and Reddaway made much of the fact that the doctors worked for the Ministry of the Interior or the KGB. Stashkin denied, however, that the KGB or the Ministry had any medical role. I asked if he had come under pressure from either body to treat particular patients in any particular way.

'I have never come under such pressure personally since I started working in the hospital in 1975. The questions of treatment and of when to discharge a patient are matters for the doctors and for the doctors alone,' Dr Stashkin insisted.

After these exchanges the visit started. We were accompanied by two guards – one a plump man who looked a little like a cartoon of the Good Soldier Schweik, and his thin partner, Muhammad. They led us through the second set of security gates into the open. The hospital buildings are grouped around a big L-shaped courtyard. To the left were most of the wards; to the right, the hospital kitchens set in a rather pretty building; ahead, ward buildings again and the workshops. A tall chimney rose at the back of one of the ward buildings. In November, it was all covered in snow. In various parts of the grounds, men were sweeping the snow away. Some of these were militia: others patients. At one end of the L-shape, there was what seemed to be a small space for sports. It had some gymnastic equipment and on the wall there was a mural of people playing games.

The windows in every building were barred. There was a great deal of barbed wire lying around the courtyard, some protecting the workshops and outside walls but much of it just dumped on the ground, derelict and vaguely menacing. But, again, the security didn't seem that stringent. There was one point at the end of the L where it didn't look as if it would be too hard to scramble out over the wall. Escapes from hospitals are not that rare. At present, the best known man on the run is Leonid Dobrov, who had organized petitions for Moldavian nationality to the Supreme Soviet. Dobrov escaped from Kishinev. Eleonora Gorbunova, Novosti's health correspondent, had been rung up a number of times by a different patient on the run who hoped for help.

The first ward we saw was the clinical ward. It is here that patients who are in some form of crisis are taken. One of the observation rooms was remarkable. Fifteen beds were crammed into one room. The beds touched and there was absolutely no privacy. It looked like a field hospital in the middle of a war except that there was no blood. Tinny music blared out of a tannoy. One man was sitting on the edge of his bed but the others were all lying down. Two men looked drugged into oblivion. The rest just lay and stared. One fidgeted by the window, irritated by our intrusion.

The patients are watched constantly by a *sanitaire*, an auxiliary nurse. The auxiliary explained, 'It's my duty to observe them. If I see the least sign of psychosis – tears, laughter, violent behaviour or the like – I call the doctor or the nurse. It's also my duty to watch them when they eat and to see that they do it without quarrelling.' The overcrowding was so bad here it seemed very likely to add to the stress patients were under.

It wasn't clear just when patients were brought into the observation room and why they were released. The rest of the ward had a number of rooms with beds in them but they were empty. At the end of the ward, there were some stained-glass panels of heroic scenes.

As was to happen in the rest of the hospital, nurses wandered outside the observation room, watching us filming. The observation room was rather grubby. Outside the ward entrance, there were buckets filled with what hadn't been eaten for dinner. Whatever the food had been, it had now been reduced to a red, stinking slop. The smell hung about unpleasantly.

Dr Stashkin denied they kept patients in isolation. They had not done so for many years. His claim flies in the face of assertions by Bukovsky and other dissidents. There was no sign of an isolation room on the wards I saw, but these were clearly the easier wards.

In theory, patients are sent to be treated, not punished. But there is no set length of time for them to be hospitalized. When they are cured or ready to be discharged to an ordinary hospital, they are sent out. Dr Stashkin insisted that the philosophy of his hospital was clinical. The aim was to cure patients. It might look like a prison but it wasn't one. Nevertheless, the atmosphere with the bars, militia and security devices is prison-like. Stashkin countered that they had a proper pattern of treatment – admission, then intensive treatment, then preparation for release. He explained that we couldn't see the admission ward or the facilities for very aggressive patients. I pressed him to explain why and he just said that it would be too difficult and disturbing for the patients.

Our arrival on the rehabilitation ward was something of an event – disturbing, perhaps, but not difficult. Patients came out to look at us.

One man put out an arm to touch Dr Stashkin. 'Do you remember me?' he said.

'Of course I remember you,' Stashkin replied.

The ward was also overcrowded. Typically, large rooms, much the size of an average sitting-room, had six to eight beds crammed into them. The laundry had been recently done. There were some nice decorations in the corridor – plants, a few pieces of art done by the patients. Dr Stashkin pointed out a sculpture called It's a Mad, Mad World and grinned. But the bedrooms themselves were much bleaker. Only one had a few decorations and personal things. In one room with six iron beds, a dragon hung from the ceiling. I was told it was because it was Chinese New Year though there weren't any Chinese patients. In another room with eight beds, there were bedside cabinets. On one there was a book for learning English. On the wall, a picture of Brigitte Bardot, the only pin-up I saw in the place. The picture had greyed with age. Clearly patients cannot make even a tiny space their own. The situation is similar to that in Broadmoor in the seventies in Britain where patients slept in large dormitories.

None of the patients I spoke to in the special hospital – and they were a restricted group – made any complaints about the conditions they were living under. It's as well to remember, though, that the ex-special hospital patients in the Serbsky had complained of many things including being robbed, injected for punishment and treated 'like a dog'.

Patients I saw unofficially were even harsher about the conditions in special hospitals. Belov said that he had seen one patient beaten by thug-like guards.

A woman who had been in Kazan Special Hospital for seven years as a result of contributing to samizdat publications said she had lived in awful overcrowded conditions usually with seven patients. There was no space between the beds. She had once been beaten when she had delivered a gift parcel to someone on another wing. It was against the rules to visit another wing. A nurse had banged her head against the door to punish her. All the other women in her cell had been deprived of privileges 'so they all had a go at me'.

No one had actually died of mistreatment but, during her time in Kazan, sixteen girls had committed suicide. She remembered one case especially. A woman had drunk toilet cleaning fluid.

The food was bad, she added, mostly bread and gruel. Three times a month they got eggs. About once a week they got meat, though it tended to be just fat. Sometimes, they got sour cream. The Kazan woman's family had also suffered. 'My family was terrorized and my sister was charged.'

Alexander Podrabinek said that relatives were often left with no information about patients. Even in these days of perestroika, they were frightened to contact groups like this, 'because the KGB might find out and that might harm the person incarcerated'. Dr Stashkin painted a very different picture. Relatives were encouraged to come, encouraged to take part in treatment. The Leningrad Hospital could be visited any day of the week other than the weekend. He didn't seem to think that exception made it hard for families.

Though patients are sent to be treated, there was much more evidence of work than of treatment. For the woman in Kazan, work was a relief. 'The sewing room was better than elsewhere because we were allowed to wash our own clothes and to watch TV.' In Leningrad, to enter the workshops isn't easy. They are guarded by large iron bars. The gate is manned by a militia man.

In the two workshops I saw, mailbags, toy sub-machine guns and also parts of audio speakers were being made. Patients seemed to handle dangerous tools; one man sliced cloth for the mailbags with a huge knife. Others who sewed the bags used scissors. In the area where they made parts for the speakers, inmates handled large hammers. Supervision seemed minimal. In each room there were two or three nurses, often elderly women.

In the corridor outside the workshop, an old, rusty machine

stands. Dr Stashkin explained it was a metal detector. But the detector was jammed up against bars so that no one could walk through it as it was placed. It seemed safe to presume it didn't work. Patients would be allowed to use such tools and machinery as few of them seem to be heavily medicated. Only a few patients had the classic look of the overdrugged. Again, it made me wonder how security is enforced.

Dr Stashkin insisted there were no disciplinary measures. When pressed, he was adamant: 'No, there aren't any.' Very aggressive patients may be excluded from the workshops but even then it would leave many who had histories of dangerousness with access to lethal tools. Dr Stashkin grinned a little smugly when I asked how that was possible. 'I expect it's because of the good relationship we have with the patients,' he purred.

On the rehabilitation ward, there is a schedule which allows little time for any treatment. Patients are responsible for keeping the ward clean: on the walls, a notice lists marks for each of the inmates for cleanliness. Two of them described the routine of their days. Neither would say why they were in. One man said that he started working after breakfast. 'I help the nurse give out the clothes to the patients when they go off to work. Then I tidy up. Then I have lunch. Then I go back to wait for the patients to return from work and then I help dress and undress them.' Another man who was sewing mailbags also said that most of the day was spent working. 'I take pleasure in my work. But this isn't home. The walls oppress me.'

The final ward I saw was a medical ward where they carry out about forty operations a year, inviting surgeons from the other Leningrad hospitals. It was completely deserted apart from a female nurse who guarded the facilities. She seemed very eager to show us the dental facilities but she couldn't open the door that led to them. Dr Stashkin became irritated at her clumsiness and I assured him I believed they did have a dentist's chair in there.

The hospital prides itself on a good record of rehabilitation. Dr Stashkin said that between 6 and 8 per cent of patients committed offences again and some did come back to Leningrad. But most stayed out of trouble and one of the pleasures of his job was receiving postcards from ex-inmates who were doing well. 'On the whole,' he smiled, 'people don't want to remember their time here particularly and so they don't stay in contact.'

I had been told that I could interview any patient I wanted. The hospital was keen to show that they did really house criminals and pressed me to talk to the murderer of blue-eyed women. He was a squat, bald man. Initially, it seemed that I was to observe the psychiatrist talking to him. The psychiatrist carried out a demonstration, jargon for a series of questions whose purpose is to get a patient to reveal his schizophrenia. It wasn't difficult, for the man was eager to talk about a project which squashed into insignificance the equation for human happiness. The bald man knew how to save mankind and create democracy. The psychiatrist handed me detailed notes that the man had written in which he accused the hospital of hampering his work by refusing to give him a personal room. How could his genius flower in such overcrowded conditions? He deserved a room of his own to study in depth. There was little doubt that he was deluded and vain but Stashkin's assistant demonstrated him with a slightly unpleasant assurance. He was using him to challenge us: so you Westerners think we have people who aren't mad in this hospital. Well, look at this. He even mentioned democracy. We let him do that. But you can see he's quite mad.

Perhaps that is unfair, for nuances are easily misunderstood in translation. It was no accident, though, that they were so eager for him to be interviewed. Yet I still had to intervene to be allowed to ask questions. Did he remember why he was here? Blankly, he said yes. He didn't offer a word of regret. The past mattered much less than his grandiose project. It was clear he was disturbed and, given his record, dangerous to release.

Even the most biased critics of Soviet psychiatry accepted that the majority of those in special hospitals were criminals with histories of violence. Indeed, it was argued that it was particularly horrific to incarcerate dissident patients with them.

The interview with the bald man ended rather inconclusively.

He continued to ramble on about his project. I didn't dispute, Dr Stashkin asked, that this person was correctly held.

I replied that the bald man did seem, on anyone's criteria, disturbed. But such cases weren't what the abuse controversy was about.

The following political prisoners were in March 1988 reckoned to be in Leningrad Special Hospital according to the Helsinki Watch Committee: Valery Gromov, Ivo Varav, Stomatislav Sudakov. They also thought a number of other people might have been in Leningrad.

At the Department of Health, I had been told I was free to see anyone that I wanted to see. Dr Egorov said, 'We have no secrets.' The Soviet side welcomed the visits of American psychiatrists to discuss cases and disagreements about particular cases. Dr Vartanyan said that when they had researched the people on the list sent by the Americans, '40 per cent were killers, criminals, etc.'. They had duped the West into taking them for persons of political significance. They had nothing to do with political dissent.' Dr Potapov, the rather flamboyant Minister of Health of the Russian Federation, promised that I could talk to anyone. I never managed to talk to Potapov again to arrange an interview for my film since he disappeared on what the Soviets call a 'komanderovski', which means literally a trip that you have been commanded to go on. But his assurances were formal.

Inside the special hospital, however, these assurances were to prove relatively worthless. The day that we arrived, I had obtained information on people on the list whom I might ask about. One was Stomatislav Grigerovich Sudakov. According to the sources at the International Association Against the Abuse of Psychiatry, Sudakov was picked up when he tried to enter the American embassy in 1974. He was charged with anti-Soviet activities and since then had been inside the special hospital system. Sudakov was on a list published by the Helsinki Watch Committee in New York and also on the IAPUP list.

When I first talked to Dr Stashkin, he accepted this. He showed me another letter from the UN Human Rights Commission which also mentioned Gromov. Stashkin complained that they got endless letters like this from interfering Westerners. He said he now had to reply to most of them.

I said on our first meeting that I would want to see Sudakov and also Gromov. Stashkin replied that if they agreed this would be possible. In order not to annoy the hospital, I had even done something I was uncertain of. During the first visit to the rehabilitation ward, a patient I didn't see slipped a letter into the palm of my hand. I didn't immediately realize what he was doing. As soon as I did, I tried to slip the letter into my pocket but my attempt was clumsy. One of the hospital staff asked politely if I had been given a letter. If so, would I give it back, as it was against the rules for inmates to hand things out to visitors. There was a proper procedure for doing so. Since I had to get back in to film, I handed the letter back.

My attempt to play by the rules didn't succeed. When I went back to film, I reminded Dr Stashkin of his assurance that I could interview both Gromov and Sudakov. I was told that I could see Gromov but that I wouldn't be allowed to film him. Thinking it was better to do that, I donned a white coat which made me look like a professional. In retrospect, I wish I hadn't. The camera crew stayed behind.

We made our way past the second set of doors and then turned up the stairs towards the ward. The ward looked much like the rehabilitation ward, except that there was a grille partitioning part of it off. The grille made that end of the corridor look like a cage. A few patients lurked behind it and stared at us. The strange salami-like smell was intense here. I asked Dr Stashkin what it was.

'It's the typical smell of mental hospitals. You smell it everywhere,' he said.

That wasn't my experience. No other Soviet hospital had that smell. The smell wasn't present even in many other parts of the Leningrad Hospital.

The ward houses some 140 patients. It was described as a diagnostic ward with active treatment. I wasn't given a tour round it but just walked up the corridor to the doctors' office. Despite the fearsome grille, here too there was some artwork.

The interview in the doctors' office must have been intimidating for the patient. There were five psychiatrists in the room. Two were the women doctors in charge of the ward. Then there was Stashkin and the Chief Psychiatrist of Leningrad. Finally, there was another psychiatrist who would be the one to interview Gromov. First, they gave me a rapid résumé of Gromov's case. Gromov was born in 1937. He was not a political prisoner at all, they claimed. He had been found guilty of trying to murder his wife back in 1974. He had been sentenced to prison but, in prison, he had become disturbed. I pointed out that he seemed to have served nearly fourteen years for attempted murder. That was an incredibly long sentence. He was being detained, I was told, no longer for the crime but because he was schizophrenic.

Gromov's detention was nearly over. Dr Stashkin explained they had told the commission which reviews cases that Gromov was in remission and should be released, initially probably to an ordinary hospital.

Then Gromov was brought in. He looked much older than fifty-one. He had a round face and grizzled grey hair. There was a bullish power in his face and, when younger, he must have looked a little like the actor, Bob Hoskins. Gromov has spent many years on aggressive wards and his appearance certainly suggests years of heavy medication. Most of his teeth are missing. His tongue wriggles out of control, one typical sign of tardive dyskinesia, a side-effect of tranquilliser use. But he looked alert and even had something of a twinkle in his eye.

The psychiatrist 'demonstrated' Gromov. The demonstration consisted of taking Gromov through a brisk résumé of his case and his political ideas. The tone was typical of many psychiatric demonstrations. The doctor isn't interested in hearing what the patient says. We know the patient is mad and the aim of this strangely ritualized dialogue is for the patient to prove to the satisfaction of the audience how mad he is by exhibiting hallucinations, delusions and utterly inappropriate ideas. Gromov sounded quite reasonable. He didn't raise his voice or act withdrawn. He accepted what the doctor put to him. Yes, he had wanted to found a Peasants' Party on Chinese lines. Yes, he had written to Brezhnev to say that and that he, Gromov, should replace him. As the psychiatrist ran through these ideas, Gromov grinned a bit, almost sheepishly. Gromov was asked if he now saw that he was ill then. 'Oh yes, I was ill,' he confirmed, a little airily.

After fifteen minutes of questioning, Yelena said that I wanted to ask questions. The psychiatrists seemed miffed by this, as if I was saying I wasn't satisfied with their questioning. Gromov said that he was in hospital before Leningrad where conditions were very bad. Here, they are OK. (This is like the Serbsky. The state of psychiatry is rotten, except in this splendid hospital where I am now). Gromov added he was a great deal younger when he had these ideas about Brezhnev. He didn't argue that he was never ill. But he would have a lot to lose by doing so. The commission has now promised he will be released soon, within a year. Clearly, it would be unwise to make unacceptable comments. Gromov added that he now has a considerable amount of money in the bank since he has had nothing to spend his invalidity pension on. He intends to buy a country house and retire. This turns out to be fact, not fantasy – yet another peculiarity of the Soviet system.

Finally, Gromov said that he was very worried by a friend of his who was a patient here and who has now emigrated to England, Nikolai Barranov. His case was taken up by Kinnock. Gromov was sure that Barranov was very ill. Is this little show of concern a deliberate, clever attempt on his part to curry favour with the doctors? Certainly they seem to nod approval when Gromov recites this litany of concern.

His final words to me when he left the room were, 'Viva Thatcher'. At this, too, the doctors smiled.

After he left, the doctors turned on me as if to ask, 'Was I convinced?' Even in remission, they insisted Gromov exhibited enough traits to show he was schizophrenic. It's hard to be sure. He talked quite appropriately. He seemed burnt out, which is not surprising given his long years inside. It didn't occur to me till I left Leningrad that it was strange he was not on a rehabilitation ward if he were being prepared for release.

I then asked if I could interview Sudakov. I was told that I could neither film him nor even talk to him. When I initially asked Dr Stashkin whether the Western accounts of his case

were true he then allowed himself a slight smirk. The require-
ments of medical confidentiality were absolutes a decent doctor
didn't tamper with. When I pointed out how bad this would
look, he agreed to give me a potted version of the history of
Sudakov.

'During a concert at the Tallinn Town Hall in 1984, Sudakov
smashed the cello belonging to cellist Chaykovskaya with an
axe. That was an old Italian cello. After that he underwent
forensic psychiatric examination in the Tallinn psychiatric hospital where he was diagnosed mentally ill and not responsible
for the offence he was charged with, and the commission
recommended sending him for compulsory treatment to a
special hospital, i.e. to our hospital. Following the court verdict
Sudakov was brought to our hospital in February 1985. As for
Sudakov's diagnosis and illness, I would like to discuss this
question – and could do so – with psychiatrists from Britain and
America who are going to come to the Soviet Union, as far as
I know.'

I asked why we were not able to see Sudakov.

Dr Stashkin said, 'Well, his current mental state does not
make it possible for anyone but his doctor to talk to him.'

Dr Stashkin then added a few extra details. Sudakov had
arrived at the concert with a political declaration, a swastika
and had shouted, 'Long live Reagan'.

Dr Stashkin then offered to show me the court record and
some clinical background. I pointed out this was paradoxical
since a second ago he had refused for reasons of confidentiality
to discuss Sudakov's history in general. Now he was offering
the most intimate details. The court record showed, however,
that he had spent time between 1983 and 1985 in Dnenprope-
trovsk. I assumed that this had been some period of hospitalization. Yelena translated that he had escaped from the hospital.

Mrs Gorbunova took the file, which seemed to show to her
how right Dr Stashkin was. By the next day – by which time
Sudakov had miraculously recovered enough to say that it was
fine for Stashkin to discuss his case – the following story could
be pieced together. The Soviet view is that Sudakov had had
signs of delusions from the age of twelve. He had not finished
vocational college. He had gone into the army but he had spent

much of his national service in army hospitals. Apparently, he had not liked being pushed around and he resisted those who tried to do so. In 1974, he married and he drove from Dnepropetrovsk with a political document which he tried to deliver to the American embassy. There was a fight with the militia and he was charged with anti-Soviet activities and also with parasitism since no one knew how he was making a living.

At the Serbsky he was unanimously found to be schizophrenic and he was sent to Tashkent Special Hospital. There he became something of a leader. He organized groups of patients and the hospital found they could not control him. He was sent even further off to Alma Ata – ironically the site of the WHO declaration which promised health for all by 2000 – where he again caused more trouble. By 1983, the official version was that his schizophrenia was in remission. Another interpretation might be that it was felt he had done his time. Sudakov was sent to Dnepropetrovsk Ordinary Hospital. He escaped from there in 1983 and made his way across the USSR to Tallinn where he went to live with his sister. Nothing Dr Stashkin said shed the least light on what had finally pushed Sudakov to make a demonstration in Tallinn.

In reality, the Amnesty story was confirmed. Dr Stashkin had adopted a slightly derisive tone throughout. He had made much of the unfortunate cello and grinned as he said that Sudakov had shouted 'Long live Reagan' as he sliced the strings. Dr Stashkin had also shown a rather maverick attitude to confidentiality, insisting on it at first, and then ignoring it entirely. All that illustrates, perhaps, is how hard Soviet psychiatrists find it to deal with political issues now everything is changing. I had been surprised at how much I had been allowed to see, but also irritated by the continuing evasiveness.

The situation of the special hospitals is clearly in flux. There seem to be no new admissions of political patients. The transfer of the hospitals to the Ministry of Health will improve conditions. Dr Stashkin said that he was sure there would now be more money for treatment, though he was worried about how they were going to handle security. There is talk now of a third kind of facility which will provide intensive treatment.

Human rights activists continue to be worried, however,

about conditions. The woman from Kazan, which has some 1,500 inmates, believes that there are still at least fifteen politicals in there. She is in correspondence with inmates and they claim that conditions have not improved at all. Recently released inmates remain unconvinced of major changes. Anatoly Makhinya who had been in Chernyahovsk revealed that patients would have 'starved' if it hadn't been for food parcels from outside. On 15 September 1988, a Lithuanian doctor and human rights activist, Algirdas Statkevicus told IAPUP (IAPUP Bulletin October 1988) that he had found the treatment both in Chernyahovsky and Tashkent special hospital 'merciless'. Sane men were detained as insane. Weak inmates or those 'torn with pain were forced, like slaves to do heavy physical labour.' He added that drugs had been used to torture people certainly in 1982. Like the Kazan patient, he alleged suicides were frequent. As late as the end of 1986, Statkevicus noticed no improvement. Podrabinek argued that in some ways the position of patients may be getting worse. He had information that subscriptions to newspapers had been cancelled thereby denying inmates one of their few pleasures. In some hospitals, the nurses had started cutting out controversial articles – especially articles on psychiatry – in case these excited the patients or gave them ideas. It wasn't that the nurses were more liberal before: there weren't any critical articles before. Podrabinek said, 'I see no indication of the regime changing and I am very anxious about the fate of people who have been in for so long.'

This issue is a vexed and important one that must not be forgotten in the enthusiasm for the 'new Russia'. Bloch and Reddaway estimated that as many as 300 to 500 dissidents a year were hospitalized, stressing that was a 'guestimate'. It seems clear that, as of December 1988 at least, there are still some 200 inside. It's hard to put a specific figure on those still remaining. The lowest figure is that of Amnesty, about thirty. The highest is that of the IAPUP, which is over 200.

The official attitude to Western inquiries about such patients is changing. Amnesty asked me to raise three cases with the Ministry of Health: Sergei Porsnikov, Gheorghe David and Alexander Nikiforchuk. Amnesty's information is that all were held on political charges at Dnepropetrovsk Special Hospital. Dr Egorov made inquiries and told me that looking back to January 1987, the hospital had held no patients with those names. 'One name is very familiar, though. Not Nikiforchuk but Nikifarouk. He has been discharged and his crime wasn't as the information says, trying to cross the Soviet border, but illegal drug trafficking.' Dr Egorov couldn't be sure if Nikiforchuk was Nikifarouk but he gave the information in good faith. I had no means of checking his claims but he certainly replied promptly and without any apparent irritation.

Another sign of official change was the much heralded visit of American psychiatrists headed by Dr Loren Roth in February 1989. They saw only about 40 patients, not 150 as had been originally planned. They insisted on seeing patients alone with independent interpreters i.e. not those provided by the Soviets. In a final press conference, the psychiatrists were notedly cagey. They accepted that they had been given unprecedented access but they complained that there had been some problems. Dr Morosov and Dr Vantakyan had been unavailable. Some patients had refused to see them. Had there been pressure. Most serious, they had not been allowed to see some important medical records because of photocopying problems.

Many of these dissidents were clearly wrongly diagnosed. Others might well have had some psychiatric history. But if they hadn't also had unacceptable political ideas, they probably would either just have stayed on the register or might have had spells in ordinary hospitals. Virtually none of them were physically dangerous, threatening to assault, murder or rape in the name of democracy. Yet they did end up in special hospitals for long periods and many still remain. Moreover, there's little sign of a generous approach by the Soviet authorities.

Neither Belov nor the woman from Kazan feel anyone has acknowledged what they went through. The woman from Kazan said, 'I feel like a non-person now. I can only get menial work. If I go to visit friends who are in hospital, the KGB ring ahead and tell the hospital I was a patient for seven years. If I go to complain to government agencies about anything, I am treated as if I'm not a proper adult.' A few times, as she assessed what seven years inside had done to her, she crumbled into silence and then pulled herself together, refusing to cry. Given the amount of psychiatry she had received without needing it, it was ironic that now, when she could have done with some counselling to help her get over her anger, there was none available to her. She could hardly trust *dispensaire* doctors if she confessed her feelings and her need to make sense of how a large part of her life had been ruined. They might well decide she had to go back in.

Such experiences suggest that any judgment of changes in Soviet psychiatry requires judicious balance. It is important to recognize the progress that has been made. Certainly, even critics like Podrabinek and Sakharov concede there is some desire to improve special hospitals and that 'politicals' no longer are sent there. But the Soviets themselves admit progress is slow. In March Yuri Reshetov told the visiting Americans that the transfer of the special hospitals to the Ministry of Health had not yet been completed and blamed 'technical difficulties'. Whatever those may be, the patients still inside must not be forgotten. The West needs to press not just for their release but for compensation and acceptable help with rehabilitation. The abuse controversy won't end till that is done.

8
Innovation and Research

The West's knowledge of Soviet psychiatric research is very sketchy. There are a few journals which appear in translation – *The Korsakov Journal* and *Soviet Neurology and Psychiatry*. The papers in them reveal some interesting points. First there is a wide spread of research. There are articles on many topics from nervous tics in Tourette's syndrome to the personality problems of young men training to work on ships for the Georgian steamship company.

The style of the research papers is odd, however. Nearly half the papers I sampled had very few statistics in them. The authors described developments in their own hospitals. In one case, a paper outlined how stuttering had been handled at the 6th Moscow hospital for children since the Revolution. Crudely put, there was too much history and too little science. Many commentators have sniped about the fetish for statistical precision in psychological sciences (Jordan 1968;). But in the Soviet literature, the lack of precision is striking. I could find little mention of methodological techniques like double-blind experiments which have evolved in the West to stop researchers influencing subjects to produce the results they want.

I don't pretend in this chapter to offer an exhaustive account of the current state of Soviet psychiatric research. I want to concentrate on four themes I found interesting: work, psychotherapy in a collectivist society, so-called aesthetic therapy and childhood schizophrenia.

The most interesting developments concern work. Up to 1960 or thereabouts, most psychiatric hospitals in Britain expected patients to do some work. It wasn't unknown for them to help with the cleaning of the wards. Many hospitals had farms. It was rare for patients to be paid a proper economic rate for the jobs they did but it was felt that they ought to contribute what they could to the running of the hospital. In the last twenty-five years, however, the situation has changed radically as the health services have become more professionalized. The farms have been sold off: cleaners do the cleaning. There is occupational therapy but it treats patients as disabled. They mainly do simple craft work. Sheltered workshops do offer outpatients work but they tend to pay poorly for menial work. Patients can't expect more.

Soviet psychiatry has a radically different attitude to work. It is seen both as therapeutic and as a social obligation. The most interesting innovations were at Kaluga Hospital, 180 kilometres southwest of Moscow.

The hospital is on the edge of the town. The first thing you notice is a building with a mural of workers' hands raised to the sky in triumph. For once the propaganda isn't a total lie, for Dr Lifschitz, its director, has presided over a successful experiment. He persuaded a local enterprise to build a hospital factory. The local Party helped, its secretary explained, 'especially because Dr Lifschitz never asks for too much money'. The hospital workshops are a serious business, not charity for the poor disabled. They build electronic components for cars, steering wheels, locks, parts of power boats. They meet real deadlines for real orders.

The workshops belong jointly to the hospital and a local factory. The doctors decide when patients are fit for work and how much they can do. The 'enterprise' is consulted. Dr Lifschitz pointed out a rota on one wall just by a bust of Lenin. Some patients worked eight hours, others worked only five. Working conditions are certainly adequate. The factory is relatively clean. Safety notices hang all over the place. The patients are given proper training. Clearly, too, there's been considerable capital investment in equipment. The head of the enterprise pointed proudly to some robots that they had just installed.

Patients work under supervision. A nurse is on duty in every workshop, wandering around in her great white hat. A doctor is in the building during working hours. Patients are expected to be punctual and efficient. Two quality controllers check every electronic component, that they produce.

This is very different from sheltered workshops. At Kaluga, the work is skilled and the workers are paid properly. Dr Lifschitz explained that most got the proper industrial wage and also some disability pension. The enterprise funded the salaries: the government the pension. There were workers who were making in the region of 400 roubles a month, very good money for the USSR.

The director of the enterprise said that initially all the business people had been very sceptical. They were worried about what it would be like to employ patients. They didn't know if it made economic sense. Also, they felt awkward because they didn't know how to behave around 'lunatics'. The awkwardness had passed. 'The workers here are at least as good as any others,' he said.

The patients at Kaluga seemed to enjoy being given the chance to do proper productive work. In the West, an experiment like Kaluga would spawn an associated host of research studies. It's a pity that there have been very few here. It would be interesting to know, for example, if patients had more self-confidence than was usual. I also wondered what the effect on family relationships was. Usually in the West if a man has a breakdown, he loses the status of breadwinner. This can lead to personality changes in family power. There was no sign of such research. Patients said that they enjoyed the work. One man explained that he didn't have much difficulty in mastering the machinery because he had done similar work before he had had a breakdown.

Kaluga has recognized that if patients can handle machinery, they deserve more responsibility in their lives. Partly with money from the factory, Lifschitz has built two hostels in which people can live. Most rooms have four beds. Here, there is room for patients' possessions. As part of hostel life, patients are prepared for their return to the community. A certain typically Soviet nannying is still in evidence. Each floor in the hostel has a nurse who has her own office and in some sense 'runs' the floor. There are no community meetings as there would be in the West to decide on household issues like what the week's menu should be. Nevertheless, the atmosphere is very different from that on most hospital wards. Patients expect to leave usually after twelve to eighteen months. They can get a flat in Kaluga and continue to work in the hospital factory.

With the advent of perestroika, Kaluga is having to change some of the financial arrangements. The disability monies paid by the State would diminish. The enterprise is confident that they could be self-financing easily. The sick workers were good workers.

Kaluga is not principally a research institution. The development of an impressive programme of work is the result of one psychiatrist's vision. It reveals the complexities of the situation that Lifschitz, who had done all this excellent work, is the same Lifschitz who incarcerated Medvedev!

The controversies about dissidents have made it easy to imagine that Soviet psychiatry is 'monolithic', with only one view allowed. Soviet psychiatrists claim this shows the ignorance of the West. Historically there have always been battles between Moscow and Leningrad with the Leningrad school generally being reckoned to be more liberal – especially given its interest in psychotherapy.

The Leningrad School

Outside the Bechterev Hospital in Leningrad, there is a massive head of Bechterev, authoritative and, of course, bearded. All Soviet institutions honour their founders in a way that would seem cloying in the West. Hospital corridors are nearly always lined with grave-looking men sporting the beard of wisdom. Notices proclaim they directed this hospital or this department of the hospital for a particular time. These monuments to the past suggest that Soviet institutions are not obsessed with the new. There's less frantic seeking for novel theories or insight than in the West. Appointments seem to depend much less than in the West on what you publish, though a good deal on who you know. This reverence for the past is reflected in the rituals of the visit. It's hard to imagine a visitor to the Maudsley Hospital in England, for example, being given a detailed historical account of the work of Maudsley as a serious introduction to the current work of the hospital that is named after him. In years of touring Soviet institutions I've never had it happen. At the Bechterev, however, the introduction is red caviar, tea and history.

In Bechterev's case, the history is interesting. He was one of the founding fathers of Russian psychiatry. He set up his Institute in 1908 well before the Revolution. The Tsar did not like him but Bechterev managed to survive. Professor Modest Kabanov, the current director, is a flamboyant man who likes to pepper his talk with quotes from Hegel, Voltaire, Rousseau and many other literary figures. He lapses into French and German phrases. He gestures frequently like a caricature of a Frenchman in an Agatha Christie book. Kabanov exudes *kultur*. He proudly pointed out Bechterev's progressive credentials. When the Revolution came, Bechterev was rewarded till, in some obscure way, he clashed with Stalin. Stalin hated all psychiatrists. Rumour has it that Bechterev either told him he was paranoid or told other people in the Party that Stalin was paranoid. Soon after this unwise diagnostic move, Bechterev died. It is now alleged that he might have been poisoned on Stalin's orders. Photographs of Bechterev's funeral show a full house. His cortège was something of a public demonstration.

Bechterev refused to see mental illness as either purely medical or biological. He stressed the importance of social and emotional factors. He gave his school a much more liberal attitude than that in Moscow. In Leningrad, for example, Freud was rarely taboo. Some of the Leningrad school's attempts to grapple with psychotherapy have been described by Lauterbach (1985) in his useful, if rather technical, book. Its previous director, Meyassechev, outlined a theory of psychotherapy which took much from the West but insisted on the therapist's right to give direct advice.

Kabanov insists on the value of this rounded approach. He prides himself on never having diagnosed anyone as a sluggish schizophrenic because he believes the diagnosis is harmful. The stigma attached would cripple someone's prospects.

The main focus of the research at the Bechterev is into rehabilitation and psychotherapy. Two wards are devoted to psychotherapy and these wards did not appear to be locked. More than most Soviet hospitals, the Bechterev aims to get patients back into the community and working. The doctors at the Bechterev coax and nag patients to get motivated to get better.

One patient was an actor who said that his only problem was that he now suffered acute anxiety about going on to the stage. He agreed to be interviewed because he felt that this would be a step forward. Irina, who complained bitterly about being on the list and the social attitudes to mental illness, said that she wanted to return to work as soon as possible.

The focus on psychotherapy showed itself in an interesting way. Irina had been previously in another Leningrad hospital. She said that the conditions in the hospital had been terrible and that she had been taken there against her will. The Bechterev was far better. She made no allegations of brutality or ill-treatment but she felt the previous hospital was brusque, dirty and unhelpful.

The staff said that before we left the ward we ought to talk to them about Irina. They didn't deny what she said, or try to suggest she was too mad to have a sensible opinion. Rather, they wanted us to have a sense of how her personality worked. She was actually a rather lazy patient. She enjoyed the goodies of care. If there were dances or outings, she was enthusiastic. But she did not like being asked to work on herself or to confront her problems. She didn't want to strive to get better. They doubted her motivation for getting back to work. Just words! It wouldn't surprise them if she started to complain about their ward if they started making demands on her. The analysis was interesting – I've no way of knowing whether it was plausible – and shows an intriguing side of the liberal tradition. It has made medical staff more willing to listen attentively to patients even though what they say can be turned against them. There wasn't, however, any ongoing research into how to avoid such dependency.

The aesthetic

Kabanov explained that much of what they offer is called either aesthetic therapy or culture therapy. This is one of the goodies that Irina liked.

In many Soviet hospitals, there is a tradition of taking patients for a walk. On the Sunday, patients were taken to Pushkin, some 100 kilometres from Leningrad. It's a magnificent palace, bedecked with golden domes and green cherubs outside. The inside is rather like a grander, even more baroque version of the Brighton Pavilion. There is a splendid ballroom covered with mirrors framed in gilt. Many of the rooms contain priceless works of art. One sitting room was lined with amber. The walls of one hall are hung with fine paintings by Poussin and other eighteenth-century masters.

Pushkin was rebuilt after the Second World War when the Nazis had occupied and destroyed it. Taking patients there shows faith in them, something few Soviet hospitals manage. It's also true that Western and Japanese hospitals would assume culture was simply beyond the ken of the mentally ill. Bingo, perhaps. But show them art and they wouldn't know what they were looking at or how to behave. They'd giggle, get bored, fractious. The public would stare at them. In Leningrad, there were none of these negative attitudes.

The patients handled the outing well. They could have been any group of visitors. Dr Khashkarov, in charge of the borderline wards, explained that they did not tell museums patients were coming because that could be counter-productive. They'd be asked why they wanted to inflict them on the museum. Sometimes when they had warned museums, they had been treated oddly or rudely.

The patients enjoyed the visit and actually concentrated. They didn't get lost in the maze of people. They listened to the guide. They occasionally even asked questions. After the visit was over, they claimed that it made them feel better. Ludmilla said that the beauty they had seen was 'uplifting'. But there's no research undertaken which either justifies such outings or examines precisely what they do achieve. It is assumed they're a good thing.

The strangeness of the outing was especially striking since the patients returned to a quite restrictive hospital setting. The Bechterev is less oppressive than most Soviet hospitals but the wards are still locked. The doctors and nurses still wear regulation white. The workshops are actually rather more oppressive than in Kaluga or even the Leningrad Special Hospital. That's largely because they are in a dark, old building. When I first reached it, a group of patients were shifting heavy sacks. Their faces were contorted with effort. In the workshops, staff didn't seem to be using research to confront what would be a pressing problem soon. The workshop director explained that they were now under pressure to become self-financing. But there had been no work done on seeing what the implications were. The director tossed out rather suddenly the fact that this meant that they might have to cut the patients' wages, the opposite of what Kaluga's calculations revealed.

Without the rigorous research, the emphasis on rehabilitation to which Kabanov often returned can't hope to be that effective. Much Western work on rehabilitation suggests that programmes have to be carefully designed and implemented. They have to be monitored if they are to help patients get back to their lives.

The Bechterev has clearly had to struggle because psychotherapy contradicts so much of the ideology of communism. Psychotherapy is individualistic. To seek to make each person whole, perfect and brimful of insight clashes with a collective ideology. What if the interests of the individual differ from those of the group? The Bechterev managed in difficult times to keep some tradition of psychotherapeutic work alive in the USSR. That remains an important triumph. But the lack of critical research means that now, when it is much more possible to promote psychotherapy, there isn't much of a scientific base to build on. In Moscow, a centre for psychotherapy is being planned. Its initial philosophy sounds like a replay of the chaotic enthusiasm for encounter groups in the sixties in the West. Dr Slutsky, who has been appointed its director and glories in the title of Chief Psychotherapist of Moscow, intends to have 'growth videos' and gimmicks sadly reminiscent of the heyday of Esalen, the American therapy centre that pioneered the encounter group and its excesses. It's psychobabble Moscow style.

The All Union Centre and childhood schizophrenia

The All Union Centre in Moscow is much more conventional than the Bechterev. Its philosophy is overtly scientific. The

Centre is part of a huge complex of medical buildings in the southeast of Moscow. The hospital decor reflects the Institute's status. Everything is lavish. There's far more space than in other hospitals. The Institute's director, Dr Yastrebov, liked to point out not just the inevitable plants but the art. The standard of the tapestries, sculptures and paintings in the wards is high. Some are the work of patients but many have been bought to give the place a certain gloss. Aesthetic therapy is fashionable here too.

Dr Yastrebov is an open, engaging man with an elegant mop of white hair. He was about to change jobs and he told his rather nervous deputy to get used to talking to journalists: once he had the top job, such contacts would be necessary. Yastrebov spread out a photo and map of the medical complex. Psychiatry was an independent Institute, of course, but linked to other facilities. There are four departments in the Institute. One for acute cases, one for geriatrics, one for borderline states and one for children. Yastrebov stressed that they were a research Institute. They tended to take patients who interested them. But regional hospitals could also ask for patients to be sent there if the Institute's 'expertise' was needed and the lowly provinces couldn't cope. Patients come from all over the USSR. Difficult cases, especially those where diagnosis wasn't easy were common, reflecting the passion for pinning down the precise degree of illness someone had. They also took 'cases who are resistant to treatment', Yastrebov smiled. By resistant, he didn't mean those who resisted or objected to treatment, but those who were not getting cured.

'It is a model Institute,' Yastrebov said. He was not being vain. The fact is that few facilities in the Soviet Union are like this with no overcrowding and impeccably clean wards. The Institute can afford to hire specialists to run particular activities, like a PE teacher for the children's ward.

'Only a socialist state could have built an Institute like this,' Yastrebov beamed with pride. Like the Bechterev, the All Union Centre is clearly a good hospital. But, again, it didn't have the liveliness of research you would find at the Institute of Psychiatry in London or New York's Psychiatric Centre.

After the initial orientation, Yastrebov strode down the first of many long corridors. He mimicked running and explained it was so long it was the only way to cope. Patients and cleaning staff both complained of the sheer size of the Centre. Yastrebov pointed out the library and the cinema. Both looked pristine but, oddly, there didn't seem to be a patient in the library. The cinema recently showed *One Flew Over the Cuckoo's Nest*, yet more glasnost in action.

The wards were all locked. Yastrebov has a master key. When he walked on to any ward, he always caused a ripple. The boss was here! Everyone looked. He first took me on to the children's ward which takes both boys and girls aged between seven and fifteen. Yastrebov showed off the many good points, a smart room for visitors, many pretty pictures, a nicely-appointed play room. He opened the fridge to show the gifts that parents bring. It was full of apples and biscuits. The ward also has two classrooms and a recreation area with a piano. Children loafed around this area and one boy was playing the piano beautifully. It was explained that he was frightened of school because there was bullying but he had no fear of music school.

The children watched us carefully. Suddenly, there was a howl of alarm from a tall, gangly boy with a moustache. He was firmly but not unkindly marched to his bedroom by a nurse. It's always hard to get an impression in a first visit, and Yastrebov rather tended to sweep me from one place to the next. There wasn't really time to do more than admire the look of the place before being taken through the corridor at one end to the autism ward.

Autism is a problem of non-communication and very hard to treat. At the Centre, they take children very early – from two or three. The families aren't involved in the treatment which is largely speech therapy. 'This is the hardest work of all,' Yastrebov said. The approach here seemed eccentric in some ways. The families are allowed to visit but they are not involved in the actual therapy. Yet Yastrebov says they succeed with 35 per cent of cases. A further 20 per cent are somewhat improved. These statistics appear to be the result of internal evaluation by the Centre staff. Again, one wished for more rigorous inquiry.

The children are clean and well looked after. They pranced around in front of the cameras. One boy edged closer, wanting to touch the equipment but, a typically autistic reaction, when offered the chance, he ran away.

Again, the curious impression remained, given the status of the Institute, that not much original research was going on. When I visited a second time, Dr Yastrebov had gone to his new job and the psychiatrist in charge, Dr Koslova, was much more pessimistic. She wasn't sure that they were getting enough cases to keep the ward open.

The Soviet Union has more of a tradition of child psychiatry than most Western countries. Dr Koslova explained that the ward took eighty-two children. Most of them were schizophrenics but there were also some with organic disorders. There were a few with borderline states. Finally, there was a group who weren't schizophrenics but had 'schizophrenic-like symptoms'. This seemed to include behaving badly. Dr Koslova listed 'maladaptation in school, strange behaviour, bad contact', the tendency to smoke and drink a lot and to be too interested in sex given their age. One of the staff's interests was to see how they could correct the behaviour of these semi-schizophrenic children. In the USSR, children who are treated as delinquents in Western countries tend to end up in hospital. Moscow has one psychiatric hospital exclusively for children with something like 1,000 beds. There is a children's hospital too in Leningrad but in some areas like the Baltic Republics there's little provision. It proved impossible to arrange to visit the Leningrad hospital.

The children at the All Union Centre are the most difficult cases.

The children who suffer from schizophrenia are not treated harshly. There's much physical affection from the staff. Even so, the children have many restrictions placed on them.

Dr Koslova, the ward director, was very welcoming when we went back to film. The children had obviously been spruced up for us. Dr Koslova explained that many of them, some as young as six, were schizophrenic. Some were born schizophrenic, she added. They had either inherited the disease or developed it on the instant of birth! Her own thesis was on this subject. She believed that about 10 per cent of schizophrenics were born with the disease. She knew of the recent research at the Middlesex Hospital in London that has claimed to identify a schizophrenia gene. It fitted in with her own view of the disease, she suggested. Gurling (1988) has been careful to state that though there may be a gene for schizophrenia, it doesn't express itself till the late teens. In the Western literature, there are controversies about whether childhood depression exists at all and, in general, the onset of schizophrenia is thought to occur round the age of fifteen or so.

Dr Koslova said there were on the ward many examples of children with this genetic defect. She patted a young boy of about seven who came from Armenia. 'A sad case,' she sighed. He came from a family of schizophrenics. His mother was schizophrenic; his father was alcoholic. The lad had no hope. She hugged him and explained that, as he misbehaved, he wasn't allowed to go out on walks. For the last two months, he had not been off the ward. Rather gently, Dr Koslova asked a boy from Georgia what he wanted. 'To get out of here,' he snapped. The tall gangly boy who had howled was still on the ward, somewhat calmer. Many of the patients, Dr Koslova said, would be back because it was impossible to cure them – and their genes.

Dr Koslova did have some precise statistics. A survey they had carried out of 225 children who had been admitted led them to believe that 1/15th (i.e. just over 6 per cent) were 'inborn schizophrenics'. They were continuing to do research in this field and they hoped to be able to offer genetic counselling – like in the West.

Like a number of psychiatrists, Dr Koslova seemed rather struck with the psychological consequences of current social changes. She said that they were seeing many children who were the victims of broken families. Many mothers were alcoholics. The children had to be kept in a dormitory because there was nowhere else. This was a bleak picture. There would be more 'bad behaviour' for doctors to manage, she seemed to suggest. Dr Koslova had no doubts, however, of the existence of schizophrenia at birth. It's ironic that Western pressure has done much to cast doubt on sluggish schizophrenia but, so far, there's very little sign of scepticism about this equally strange diagnosis.

It's sad to report that even at the All Union Centre there were problems related to filming and politics. Dr Yastrebov had warned that by the time we came to film he would have moved on to his new job. The arrangements for filming had been agreed in the presence of his deputy who was to be the new director. These arrangements, however, didn't turn out to bind the hospital. When we returned to film, the deputy said that we could not film any patients. He announced that, 'Our decision is final'.

I protested, as did Yelena and Eleonora Gorbunova. One doctor said they feared that filming would provoke psychotic episodes in patients. That had often happened.

'How many times have your patients been filmed?' I asked.

'Never,' he admitted.

'So how do you know? I've filmed many patients and there's never been a psychosis.'

In the middle of the row, the deputy disappeared out of the room. He returned a few minutes later. It then turned out that the real director of the hospital was someone quite different, a Dr Tiganov. Dr Tiganov lived in an office at the side of the acute ward. Had Dr Tiganov been there all the time that Yastrebov was apparently the director? Tiganov turned out to be an ex-student of Snezhnevsky and a firm believer in sluggish schizophrenia. But he accepted that we had reached an agreement to film and that it would look bad for the hospital to renege on that.

Nevertheless, on both the acute and geriatric wards, our filming was very restricted. We were allowed to interview only one patient – a thin man who said that he was frightened 'of everything' and had just been brought on to the acute ward for the third time. It was hard to work out just why he should be of any research interest.

After this long period of little contact, the West needs to know much more about innovation and research in the Soviet system. Until the dissident debate, it was accepted that in the provision of certain services – access to polikliniks, those for the chronically handicapped (Wing 1977) – the Soviets had much to offer. Today, I would argue that is especially true in the area of the constructive use of work. There is also much the Soviet Union could learn from our psychiatric practice, flawed though it might be, especially that patients have a voice and ought to be heard. The obsession with biology and organic causes may be as much of an obstacle in the development of good care as any political repression. It is those organic ideas, so evident on Dr Koslova's ward, which make it easy for patients to be seen as damaged and, as a result, unfit to have a voice.

Freud argued long ago of the need to involve the patient in a 'therapeutic alliance'. As pressure groups like MIND have campaigned in the West for better rights for patients, Freud's notion has penetrated into many parts of the psychiatric system. British hospitals regularly hold ward meetings in which patients discuss how the ward is run. In New York, groups of social workers like those in Project Reach Out, who offer the homeless mentally ill on the streets the chance of care, talk about the need to 'engage' the patient. It would be absurd to suggest that Western psychiatric practice is democratic but it is becoming less high-handed at least in many places. There's absolutely no sign of that in the USSR.

Finally Marx, the ideological father of the Soviet Union, whose statue rises all over the place, would be quite amazed by the continuing, absolute faith in biology. If he were to return from Highgate to a Soviet hospital, he would be appalled by what is being passed off in the name of his theory.

9

The Commission Hearings

One of the most interesting innovations in the new liberal climate has been the new role of commissions of psychiatrists. In this chapter I want to examine their working.

It would be wrong to suggest that such commissions were set up by the new law of January 1988. Even in Stalinist times, psychiatrists were meant to review cases of detained patients every six months. In theory, a patient could appeal to a commission to examine his case.

In practice, however, the commissions were ineffective. Few patients asked them to intervene. Moreover, there was no appeal from the decisions of the commission. The January 1988 law defined the procedures under which patients could appeal if they were not satisfied.

Some critics like Andrei Sakharov have welcomed these new regulations suggesting that they have considerably improved the situation. Others, like Podrabinek, remain sceptical.

Dr Tichonenko, the Chief Psychiatrist of Moscow, is a plump man with a rather shy grin. Like Dr Kosirev, he wanted to know what my views were before we got down to discussing access. Tichonenko has recently moved into his post. He has argued that Moscow's services badly need to encourage patients to come voluntarily to seek help. Psychiatry should be loved, not feared. He has written that (1988) 'The question of the democratization of psychiatric aid concerns mostly the people afflicted with marginal neural and psychic disorders like neurosis and depression.' Tichonenko acknowledged that many of these didn't need 'dynamic clinical attention'. Or forced treatment. 'Such people must have the opportunity to apply for a specialist's consultation only when they wish so themselves as is the case with physicians, surgeons, oculists and other doctors.'

Dr Tichonenko is seen as a liberal and he was not the least defensive. He explained that it wouldn't be easy to film the commission at work. Much of the material was confidential. I easily accepted that. In Britain, it would have been very difficult to arrange to film Mental Health Review tribunals which review the cases of detained patients. After some negotiation, Tichonenko agreed that, though he and his colleagues were nervous of exposure, I could film. The only proviso was that patients accepted it freely.

As Chief Psychiatrist of Moscow, Dr Tichonenko supervises the whole region's psychiatric system. He sits as chairman of the commission patients appeal to. He explained that in Moscow there were 200,000 patients on the register. Many did not want to be on it but there was a limit to the number of cases the commission could review. They saw six to eight cases a week. The procedure had to be thorough. When a patient wrote to request a hearing, they would assign one doctor to examine the patient's record, delving through the paperwork. In general, that took a month. A representative of the *dispensaire* that opposed release would be asked to appear before the commission.

In Britain or in America, similar hearings involve lawyers. The patient has the right to be legally represented. Western tribunals are not composed solely of doctors and recognize that decisions concerning potentially dangerous patients aren't solely medical. Questions such as whether a community should take the risk of release have nothing to do with psychiatry. In addition, patients can call witnesses to testify about their behaviour in the outside world.

Even under the new law, Soviet procedures reflect the continuing power of psychiatrists. They are judge, jury and expert witness. No other profession is involved.

The commission hearings I attended were at the 14th *dispensaire* in Chekhov Street. They were held in what would have been the ballroom, a splendid setting. A huge table for twenty people was on one side of the room. Twelve psychiatrists sat, reviewing the papers, seven men and five women. Cynically, I wondered if this magnificent muster of medical personnel was routine. Did they use twelve when there was no filming?

Tichonenko chaired the meeting and took the leading role in questioning the patients. The cases I witnessed were those of a woman in her early fifties called Valentina and a man of much the same age called Vladimir.

At the start, the patient was not there. The panel of psychiatrists first heard the doctor who had examined the paperwork read out a letter in which Valentina requested a hearing. The letter said that Valentina now felt well enough not to need to be on the register.

Then the doctor from Valentina's *dispensaire* outlined the reasons why she thought it inadvisable to release Valentina. The doctor was a little nervous but assembled a lengthy case against her patient, going back to 1964. 'She has thyroid problems,' the doctor started. Valentina had had an operation on her thyroid gland but that had left her listless and tearful. It had also been the trigger for a series of mood swings which 'made her either extremely active or deeply depressed'. Valentina was first put on the register in 1964. Then, she was admitted to the Kashenko for the first time. But 'when she was released her condition was not particularly good'. The doctor added that there had been a suicide attempt too. The doctor did not mention any incident in which Valentina had been violent to others so it's reasonable to suppose that there was none. The doctor wound up insisting that it was too risky to remove Valentina from the register.

Valentina then entered the room. She had not, of course, heard the case against her. Valentina was a heavy woman with blonde hair. She had tried hard to look good; she wore much rouge and had been to the hairdressers. She was nervous, not surprisingly in the face of twelve doctors, but she composed herself. As she sat down, she smoothed her dress and folded her hands. She appeared calm as she began to face what can only be called an interrogation. Dr Tichonenko made little attempt to put her at her ease. I had experienced him as a courteous, twinkling man, but this was a different persona, as a transcript of what happened shows:

Dr Tichonenko: You were treated and observed . . . until 1982–3. So over a period of almost twenty years you've been seeing psychiatrists, you've been in mental homes and at the *dispensaire*. How do you explain all this?

Valentina: The first time I came to see the psychiatrist it was quite unexpected. I didn't know what it would lead to. But my eyes don't roll about, my arms and legs don't tremble. I don't feel anxiety pangs as I used to after taking pills and . . . a doctor, whom I saw privately, warned me, and said if you can bear the strain of not taking pills over this period then it will be okay, because you've got used to them. Well, now I don't take anything . . .

Dr Tichonenko: A few more questions. During these twenty years that you were seeing psychiatrists, how many times were you in psychiatric hospitals?

Valentina: At first, often.

Dr Tichonenko: All together, how often?

Valentina: Well, I haven't counted. Maybe, about five times – but that was only at the very beginning. Maybe you think that's an awful lot, but you should take into account that I used to go voluntarily . . .

Dr Tichonenko: That's precisely what I want to stress, that you felt something that prompted you to seek help . . .

Valentina: Well, they told me that perhaps I didn't have schizophrenia – that I learnt later . . .

Dr Tichonenko was clearly annoyed that Valentina had raised this topic. He snapped, almost shouted, 'We're not discussing your diagnosis but your condition and your capacity to work. Did you have other disorders during that time?'

Valentina now began to get embarrassed. She started to suppress a giggle. She pulled herself together to explain that about a year later the atmosphere at home was bad and 'I became neurotic and had obsessive thoughts'. A particular phrase kept going through her head, she said.

'What's that?' asked Tichonenko.

'I became misanthropic.' She added, 'I feel ashamed to talk about . . . I can't go on.'

One of the women doctors told her to calm down. Valentina laughed a little more, then explained that she felt like, 'I hated everyone on earth. They were repulsive to look at . . . offensive. I felt these feelings were orders coming from a witch – about hating people.'

'So that was the phrase that kept coming into your head?' Tichonenko asked.

'I knew it had no relevance to me,' Valentina said.

'But did you try to fight it?' he demanded.

Valentina explained that she had and the method of her struggle. 'I would put on a white robe, sit in front of a mirror and imagine that the reflection in the mirror was the patient and I was the doctor and I would try to instil the idea into the person that she shouldn't worry.'

'Did that help?'

'For a while after I did that I felt high but afterwards the phrase returned.'

'I see,' said Tichonenko. He made no attempt to reassure her.

It's important to recall that this witch-like symptom had afflicted Valentina years ago. She was describing the early years of her illness in the sixties. Yet it was to count against her now. Having explored the witchery, Dr Tichonenko handed over to one of the other doctors, who had spent most of the time with his head buried in the file, flicking over pages while Valentina talked. His manner was more gentle.

Doctor: Is your mood all right today?
Valentina: Well, I'm nervous . . .
Doctor: No, I mean your mood.
Valentina: Of course, I can't say I've succeeded in everything or that I'm completely hopeless. After all, I'm coping . . .
Doctor: And when you feel low, is it worse than your mood today?
Valentina: When I'm upset . . . well, I think every person when upset . . . they feel they're in a dead-end . . .

The doctor seemed satisfied. A third doctor then intervened. He was a burly man who frequently jabbed his finger for emphasis. He wanted to know if Valentina was good at differentiating what caused her feelings. She had had periods of depression, anxiety and obsessive thoughts, 'but you also alleged that you had experiences resulting from the effects of drugs when your eyes rolled and you had inner anxieties and tremors' – he gestured, allowing his hand to tremble – 'could you tell what resulted from your illness and what from the drugs?'

'Yes I could,' Valentina promised.

'You could – yes?' He remained dubious.

'I've come to the doctor and returned the drugs,' she pointed out. The offending drugs were sent back.

'So they had a bad effect?'

She said they had. That was the end of what must have been a very difficult interview for her. Valentina was asked to wait outside in the corridor for a few minutes. Again, the proceedings would become secret.

Tichonenko then went round the table basically soliciting a vote on her sanity. In general, the psychiatrists felt she had proved her case. Most argued that she should be taken off the register and encouraged to go for active treatment. One man doubted that she would be sensible if she started to have one of her mood swings. 'I don't agree that she will come to us if she feels ill. She didn't come when she drank luminal.' She had only been saved then because her parents had been alive. Now they were dead.

Tichonenko summed the case up, saying that he didn't think that Valentina was in an active phase, 'but she shows residual signs which are personality changes of a schizophrenic type. It's impossible not to notice them. We don't have the right to say that she has come out of her illness and has recovered her personality and all her abilities. That would be definitely a mistake.' The witch's tale and her giggling proved that.

Nevertheless, he felt, as was clearly the mood of the meeting, that keeping her on the register was no longer justified. Valentina was called back into the room. She looked very nervous. Tichonenko asked her to sit down. It soon became clear that, though she had won her release, she wasn't to think that she was really cured. Again, his tone was severe and worth quoting in full; he told Valentina: 'Valentina Vasilyevna, we have thoroughly looked at your case in all its details and have come to the following conclusion. Your request is granted and you can be taken off the list. But you understand we wouldn't like to part on this note, because after all as doctors we cannot but recognize that you have had certain mental disorders. Your condition today is not optimal and therefore, in taking you off the list, we are not refusing to give you help in the future if you request it. From now on there will be no mandatory calls to come to the *dispensaire*, no mandatory consultations or treatment will be proposed. But we hope that you will be sensible about your own health. If you feel your capacity to work declines, if obsessive ideas return, if you feel low and have abrupt changes of mood and aggravated feelings of resentment, you can come to the *dispensaire* without being put on the list and you will receive treatment. You can even be hospitalized if you wish in the open sanitorium ward of our hospitals, in any one of them.'

Valentina asked, 'What about work?'

Tichonenko said, 'With work, you solve your problems without the interference of psychiatrists and also now without the help of psychiatrists. If you need a clearance card from work, they will say you are not on the list.'

Valentina said thank you with only a hint of a smile. The whole experience had been gruelling. The *dispensaire* doctor left too but he didn't speak to Valentina.

The second patient was much more pathetic. Vladimir attended dressed in a faded blue suit on which he had pinned his many war medals. He carried himself stiffly. He looked pale and used a walking stick to support himself. It was a surprise to hear that this slightly wooden lame old man was not just on the register but on the special register as he displayed aggressive tendencies. Again, Tichonenko dominated the questioning.

Having referred to this special register for extreme aggression, Tichonenko demanded, 'How are we to understand this?'

Vladimir retained his wooden look. 'I never wrote against anyone or threatened anyone.' He didn't seem fit enough to be a social menace.

'What sort of conflicts did you have with your wife?' asked Tichonenko.

'Well, I sometimes argued with my wife. You see, there were two women, my wife and mother-in-law. I was in the minority. My mother-in-law also drank. Then it seems they wrote against me,' Vladimir said.

'Did you know that she was seeing her relatives?'

It seemed that this was one of those cases in which relatives had been the prime movers.

Tichonenko was not as sharp as he had been with Valentina. He wanted to know if Vladimir's place of work knew about the register.

'I'm very open about it,' Vladimir said.

None of the other doctors were interested in raising other aspects of the case. Vladimir was told to go. He shuffled out using his cane and carrying his battered briefcase. It was typical, Tichonenko said later, for patients to arrive wearing their regalia of medals. It did Vladimir no good.

Vladimir was sent out to wait for his verdict but there was much less discussion than with Valentina. None of the doctors argued that he ought to be removed from the register though there was no evidence that he had actually been dangerous. When Vladimir was brought back he was never told what their decision was. Rather he got a lecture on how he took his medicines.

The doctors passed a large book around the table for signature, which recorded their decision. As they were doing so, the doctor who had asked Valentina if she could differentiate her own emotions from those caused by drugs jabbed his finger again. 'I have a question not related to your health,' he told Vladimir. 'Do you keep your medicines properly? Has the *dispensaire* told you how to look after them?'

There hadn't been any suggestion earlier that Vladimir didn't take the drugs properly. He had come well prepared, however, for he took out of his briefcase a plastic bag containing all his supply of drugs.

'Yes,' he told the doctors. The bag was evidence in his favour, surely, as a methodical drug taker.

'Do you take them properly?' asked the doctor.

'Yes.'

'Before or after meals?'

'I take them before and after meals,' said Vladimir.

'Why before and after?' demanded the doctor.

Vladimir repeated that he took the drugs as the doctor ordered. To prove the point, he handed his pharmaceuticals bag to Dr Tichonenko who didn't open it but passed it round to the left. It was an extraordinary scene, the psychiatrists staring at this bag.

It didn't, however, lead to Vladimir being given any official decision.

The jabbing doctor boomed: 'We've talked about this amongst ourselves and we think that you should stop taking medicines orally . . . it would be better to have injections once a fortnight, because to take so much in your stomach could lead to complications such as gastritis and so on. You've been on them too long and I would suggest that you have injections instead.'

That was the end of the commission as far as Vladimir went. He shuffled out again, disappointed but, to my surprise, not angry.

Dr Tichonenko may have been harsh in questioning patients but there's no doubt that his commission is a proper inquiring body. It doesn't provide a whitewash. Dr Tichonenko said that they often found *dispensaires* had been too conservative. As Chief Psychiatrist, he also saw the commission's brief as a wide monitoring one. In two cases, they had been so appalled by the way *dispensaires* handled cases that they had more or less put them on probation. He had the right to supervise any facility in the Moscow region. He reminded me that Potapov's ministry had in 1987 made stringent criticisms of the Moscow psychiatric system. Dr Tichonenko clearly sees the function of his commission as educative. Some psychiatrists did have problems adapting to the new law and 'democratization'. There were good and bad reasons, he insisted. The bad reason was fear of change. The good reason was that they were worried, as I had seen in their discussion of Valentina, about patients who might not have the insight to seek help when they needed it. He wasn't in the business of taking risks but there had been too much caution.

The commission remains very much a secret tribunal. I don't mean to cast it as a sinister body, but the rules that should apply to equitable tribunals didn't apply to it. It doesn't have to explain to patients why the doctors decide not to release them. Dr Tichonenko said that, of course, they often tried to tell patients, but it wasn't a requirement.

One indication of the fairness of any tribunal system is how easy it is to appeal against its decisions. The new law of January

1988 established that right very clearly. I was told that it cost a mere 12 roubles to get a lawyer in to advise if a patient or his family was unhappy. In the capitalist West, lawyers would cost much more. Yet despite this, there were few cases that went to court. Dr Tichonenko told me that there had been only four in the period between March and November 1988. Given that there were 200,000 patients on the register in Moscow, given that the 14th *dispensaire* alone reported six patients as being violently unhappy at its decision to release them, four cases seems a puny figure. It illustrates how unused Soviet citizens are to using the courts to press for their rights.

Vladimir had been treated peculiarly. It could be argued that he wasn't given a very sympathetic hearing and certainly that he had not been told what the panel's decision was. These would all be in the West reasonable grounds for appeal. A Western Vladimir would probably not have been satisfied. Despite his treatment, Vladimir said that he probably wouldn't appeal. He was a phlegmatic personality, he added.

Critics like Podrabinek don't believe such commissions make a difference. It is certainly easy to pick holes in the procedures. There also seems to be no concept of using lawyers at this stage to help patients present their case. Nevertheless, the new stress on commissions is a step in the right direction. And that the courts, to go by the small record so far, don't act as rubber stamps. It would be churlish of the West not to recognize that. Dr Tichonenko said that they had won two and lost two of the cases that went from them on appeal to the court.

'Fifty fifty,' he smiled, with that twinkle he had had when we discussed filming but which he never seemed to show patients.

10

The World Psychiatric Congress and After

The Congress of the World Psychiatric Association in Athens in October 1989 is likely to have to vote on whether to readmit the Soviet Union. In this chapter, I want to examine the arguments for and against their readmission. I want to suggest that it's important that the debate be constructive and generates a better deal for patients all over the world.

The run-up to the World Psychiatric Congress has been marked by intense political activity. Throughout 1988, Soviet psychiatrists explored on what terms they might be invited to rejoin the Association. In January, they welcomed a delegation from the International Helsinki Federation. Professor Stefanis, the Greek President of the WPA, visited Moscow on a number of occasions. In November, the Soviet Association of Psychiatrists passed a resolution which set up a committee to explore re-entry. Early in 1989, it welcomed a delegation of American psychiatrists who were given the chance to interview any dissident patient they wanted. Previously, there had always been controversies surrounding such visits because there were no independent interpreters, or patients had not been warned. This visit concluded without the Americans pronouncing on whether the changes in Soviet practice satisfied them. They had only seen some 40 patients. Their caution reflected the considerable importance that had come to be attached to their report. The criticisms the Americans made at their final press conference suggested that they hadn't been able to make a decisive evaluation.

As I argued in Chapter Three, there has been considerable progress on the treatment of dissidents. Hardly any are being taken into hospital now. There have been many releases. Two serious problems do remain – a group of perhaps 200 known dissident patients still detained and the question of how to rehabilitate many men and women who have been unjustly detained.

The committee of the Soviet Psychiatric Association to negotiate re-entry was chosen with some delicacy. Its chairman is Professor Modest Kabanov of the Bechterev who is head of the international section of the Soviet Association. Kabanov, with his love of quoting Hegel, Voltaire and others, has been untainted by allegations of abuse. Rather curiously, Peter Reddaway in a document circulated in IAPUP refers to him as someone with 'very little power'. Georgy Morosov is no longer the President of the Soviet Association. His successor, Nikolai Zharikov, is slightly more conciliatory and doesn't have years of controversy at the Serbsky behind him. Furthermore, no Western psychiatrists have complained of Zharikov's quoting them out of context. Vartanyan, will clearly be involved in the negotiations too but he is exclusively a research scientist, as he is quick to point out, and has 'never seen a patient. I am a biological psychiatrist.' He was in no position to sign a detention order on anyone. It seems certain that the USSR Ministry of Health has helped arrange this more 'moderate' delegation.

It isn't just the Soviets who want to re-enter. There are powerful forces within the World Psychiatric Association that want them back in. Even Sidney Bloch told me that it was a pity that 25,000 psychiatrists, 'most of them innocent', were excluded from world psychiatry. Many Third World psychiatrists have always wondered why there was such a fuss about political abuse. The voting structure of the WPA is complicated, depending on a mixture of the number of psychiatrists a country has and the dues it pays. There have been recent changes. Some Soviet psychiatrists believe that they don't have to make any concessions because the Third World and socialist bloc will vote them back in. They feel, moreover, that they have a powerful ally in the Greek president of the WPA. Stefanis ruled out of order a debate on how Gorbachev was dealing with the issue of psychiatric dissent. This debate was to be held at a regional meeting of the WPA in Washington. Stefanis said that it would be inappropriate to allow it. In April, an Executive meeting of the WPA 'provisionally' allowed the

Soviets to rejoin. The Executive doesn't have the power to let the Soviets rejoin without a vote in Congress so this was seen as another pro-Soviet manoeuvre. The real decision lies with the full WPA meeting.

Powerful interests would like it to be business as before with the USSR. At present drug companies export well under 5 million dollars' worth of medicines. There is a huge potential market there for anti-depressants and tranquillizers. In an earlier chapter, I quoted at some length from *The Pictorial Language of Schizophrenics*. The publishers of this lavish work were the drug company, Sandoz. They financed four volumes of this publication whose scientific value is unproven but whose authors control the commanding heights of Soviet psychiatry. Professor Modest Kabanov has been negotiating with a Danish firm to carry out clinical trials for drugs in Leningrad. This would be very useful for Western companies as Soviet regulations on drug trials are not as tight as Scandinavian ones.

There are some projects that would have once been considered quite surreal. Kabanov told me that there was a proposal from an American medical facilities company to build a hospital in Leningrad. Western patients would fly there where they would receive his rehabilitation therapy together with the aesthetic uplift of splendid views of the Neva River and tours of the Hermitage and other museums. High *kultur* and hard currency would bloom! Kabanov wasn't slow to get political mileage out of the proposal. 'And why would they want to build a hospital in the land of the Bolsheviks if it were true that we corral sane people into lunatic asylums?' He smiled his clever smile.

Groups like IAPUP (The International Association Against the Political Abuse of Psychiatry) fear that such pressures will combine to allow the Soviets back in without any conditions. They think that would be politically unwise. For some of those who were detained either in prison or in hospital, the issues are more personal. Some of them have called for trials of psychiatrists. Dr Koryagin has suggested that some such tribunal is necessary. The fury of some dissident circles can be gauged from some informal notes circulated to some members of

IAPUP. They refer to Morosov as 'ignorant': to Zharikov as his 'clone': and to Morosov's 'henchmen'. Their tone is exceptionally vitriolic.

Podrabinek is sceptical and wants strong guarantees but nothing like trials. He outlined to me his conditions.

I think that the Soviet Psychiatric Association should be accepted only after it has fulfilled three definite conditions. First, all political prisoners must be released, or prisoners incarcerated in mental hospitals for their religious activities. That's the first and indispensable condition. Secondly, Soviet lawyers and psychiatrists and the government must acknowledge that a system existed in which political opponents of the Soviet regime ended up in psychiatric hospitals. A public acknowledgement and public repentance of this can to a certain degree guarantee us against such a system recurring in the future. And the third condition which I think is absolutely essential is that the government must acknowledge the right of public organizations to monitor the use of psychiatry in such cases as the compulsory hospitalization or incarceration into special mental hospitals.

I think that Stefanis will not accept such conditions, but I hope common sense will prevail in the World Psychiatric Association.

Unfortunately Podrabinek didn't expand on the nature of his monitoring agency. Presumably, it wouldn't include professionals other than psychiatrists.

There's an interesting analysis behind the refuseniks who don't want the Soviet Union to rejoin. They argue that conservative Soviet psychiatrists have been told that their future depends crucially on whether they can get the Soviet Association back into the World Psychiatric Association. 'Failure,' noted Reddaway, 'would probably induce the politicians to remove them from power and, with more decent leaders installed, admit to past political abuses as the surest way of getting back into the WPA.' He added that if the Association managed to get back in at this stage 'that would be a heavy blow for the reformers'.

Not all Soviet human rights activists share this perspective, which sees all dissidents as victims of an oppressive psychiatry. Andrei Sakharov upset many others when he hinted at the Woodrow Wilson Centre that while there had clearly been political abuse, 'a serious crime on the part of the system', it was important to accept there had been 'a change for the better'. Sakharov added too that in his experience many of the dissidents had been mentally unstable. His personal impression was 'the vast majority of people of this kind I have encountered were not mentally healthy. That's my personal experience which is unlikely to be representative of the global picture if only because mentally ill people are abnormally persistent, maniacal, so to say. An abnormally large number of such individuals sought contact with me and consequently there was a considerable proportion of mentally unhinged people round me'. He stressed that this didn't excuse political abuse but, not surprisingly, he did not demand the show of repentance from psychiatry others want.

Sakharov stressed it was important to know whether the reforms would be lasting. 'Maybe it is merely window dressing. We need more detailed information. Before Western psychiatrists decide to restore Soviet psychiatry to their good graces, they need to form a pretty good idea of how things really are.' Sakharov wanted to see 'broad on-the-spot inspections'. The West should demand 'an expansion of contacts, and hope that glasnost will facilitate the information-gathering process'.

The tone of Sakharov's remarks angered many dissidents. They may reflect his own irritation at having been plagued by human rights 'groupies'. But it's impossible to dismiss his views – given his stature.

The British Royal College has passed a resolution that is much tougher in its demands. It states that Soviet psychiatry should only be let in after all dissident patients have been freed and after the Soviets have *dissociated* themselves from abuse. Bloch, who was crucial in framing the resolution, said that the term *dissociation* was deliberately vague. But, clearly, it did require the Soviets to accept that there had been some regular abuse, if not a policy. Otherwise there'd be nothing to dissociate from.

Both these conditions assume there was a policy and this, as we have seen, Soviet psychiatrists are quite unwilling to do. Professor Zharikov said, 'But we don't want to join the Royal College.'

Kabanov was liberal but not apologetic. He waved a letter

from America and said that he was going there to discuss these issues. 'But if Western psychiatrists want us to apologize, to do, if you will pardon the ballet term, a *pas de deux* or a *pas de trois*, we're not going to do it.' He bared his breast and added, 'If they want us to say we were guilty, well, we are not going to do it.' He added that in his forty years in Leningrad he had seen many mistakes but never a sane person sent away to mental hospital. 'Perhaps Leningrad is a special city,' he smiled.

Vartanyan also asserted that the conditions were humiliating. They were an 'insult to our feelings of professional responsibility'.

Sidney Bloch said he didn't want to humiliate anyone but that it was important for Soviet psychiatry to change its leaders. He thought it 'invidious', though, to name names. Other critics in IAPUP believe that the Soviet Union is so desperate to get back that they will finally accept tough conditions either for 1989 or certainly for 1995.

This politicking is interesting but those who care passionately about this issue risk losing sight of the larger context. I've argued that it is Soviet politicians who have forced changes on Soviet psychiatry. Western political pressures will also make it hard to keep the Soviet Association out of the World Psychiatric Association unless a major new scandal is revealed. The Republican administration in Washington and the Conservative government in Britain have agreed to go to a human rights conference in Moscow. Both are bastions of the right and have criticized the USSR on human rights endlessly. It really does seem unlikely that the world's psychiatrists (far less committed on this issue than President Reagan was or Mrs Thatcher is) will demand more of the Soviets.

But given the anxiety of the Soviets to get back in, there still can be negotiations.

It seems, however, perfectly possible to keep pressing for a number of points. First, all dissident patients still held must be freed and offered both financial compensation and a rehabilitation programme. Second, echoing Sakharov, it is important to institute regular exchange visits so that we remain well informed of the state of Soviet psychiatry. Third, Podrabinek's suggestion of a monitoring agency would seem to have considerable merit. It would guarantee that the abuses of the past aren't repeated. With that in place, there would be less need for some form of 'dissociation' with the past which, frankly, would only be a form of words. Podrabinek thought such an agency should cover just admission to special hospitals and compulsory hospitalization. Its brief should be wider. In Britain, for example, there has been some regret that the Mental Health Review Commission can only deal with detained patients and their conditions. It can't really comment on the state of hospitals and the treatment of voluntary patients.

There is some framework for creating such a monitoring agency. The August 1988 United Nations document, to which the Soviet Union is a signatory, already requires that countries set up a multi-disciplinary agency to which patients can complain. As a sign of good faith, Soviet psychiatrists should be asked to help set up such an agency immediately. Unlike the commissions, it wouldn't be run by psychiatrists. It would not have to be since its purpose would be to provide information rather than treat patients.

Whatever the outcome

Whatever the outcome of the debate, it seems clear that the relationship between Soviet psychiatry and the rest of the world will change. There will be far more contact than there has been for the last twenty years. It is extremely important that the West doesn't just assume that it has to teach the 'backward' Soviets. As Wing observed, there are areas in which the Soviets have something to offer – the way they care for the chronically mentally ill, for example. I have argued that, in the West, patients' ability to work isn't taken seriously, perhaps because capitalist societies find a pool of unemployment useful. In the Soviet Union patients' work is regarded as real. We have many things to learn from Soviet practices such as those in evidence at Kaluga. Trade unions and commercial enterprises have found that it's possible for disabled people to work productively and be paid properly. It doesn't seem likely that perestroika, which includes among its aims that of making commercial enterprises self-financing, will alter those attitudes. There are two other areas where lessons can be learned – the growth of 'clubs' like Transmash, and the ability of the *dispensaire* system to integrate care in the community. That integration doesn't depend on the continued existence of the hitherto massive register.

The isolation of Soviet psychiatry has clearly contributed to many of its problems. Many psychiatrists there want to see what is happening in the West because they feel they have suffered from being cut off. The West needs to capitalize on that eagerness. It should invite psychiatrists – and a wide range of them. Many Soviets complained that it was always the same top doctors who obtained the perk of trips abroad. Even if the Soviets refuse to give all the guarantees various groups in the WPA want, Western psychiatrists should encourage more contacts. They provide a chance to argue for human rights improvements, and to show that it's possible to deal with 'dangerous' patients without restricting the liberty of millions. Given Parchomenko's research on how the poor image that Soviet officials had of dissidents affected their behaviour, such contacts seem vital – and should involve professional groups often their psychiatrists too. Clearly, the climate of such exchanges will be much improved if the Soviet Union gives proper guarantees. If it doesn't, then psychiatrists who visit the Soviet Union will have always to insist on making human rights issues a central focus of any visit. That doesn't mean that there can be no discussion of scientific and therapeutic issues, but these will have to be undertaken within that human rights context. There has been enough evidence of change to justify far more contact than there has been since the late 1960s.

Finally, can patients in the rest of the world gain anything from the controversy? The Soviet situation has been an extreme and particular case of patients being denied their proper rights. In much of the Third World, too, the situation is bleak. Many patients there could do with precisely the kind of monitoring agency that Podrabinek is demanding for the Soviet Union. In the Third World, there are no organizations fighting for patients' rights. In Japan and other Asian nations, too, few such organizations exist. In Britain, America and many parts of Western Europe, there *are* pressure groups that campaign for patients' rights. Often, however, they are poorly funded. Some of the safeguards which it has been suggested Soviet psychiatry should offer would be extremely useful in other countries. In a very frank review of the *Dispatches* film in the *British Medical Journal*, Robinson (1989) wondered how good British hospitals would look to a Soviet audience. *Social Work Today* asked if the British government should apologize for its policies towards patients in the 1930s?

The United Nations document of August 1988 makes it plain that patients in many parts of the world need protection from rather arbitrary diagnoses and poor conditions of treatment. It is clear that the situation in the Soviet Union needs monitoring. So, too, does the situation in many other parts of the world. It would be useful if the continuing debate about Soviet psychiatry pushed the United Nations into making the protection of patients' rights a priority, as the 1988 document suggests it should be. What has happened in the Soviet Union reinforces the evidence from much of the rest of the world. The delicate and imprecise nature of its task and its boundaries makes psychiatry very vulnerable to abuse. Psychiatry is too important to be left to psychiatrists alone.

References

Amnesty International (1980): *Prisoners of Conscience*: Quartermaine.

Babayan, E. A., Morosov, G., Morkovkin, V. M., Smulevich, A. B. (1982), *The Pictorial Language of Schizophrenics*. Moscow: Sandoz Ltd.

Bloch, S. and Reddaway, P. (1977), *Russia's Political Hospitals*. London: Gollancz.

(1984), *Soviet Psychiatric Abuse*. London: Gollancz.

Bukovshy, V. (1978): *To Build a Castle*. London: Deutsch.

Cohen, D. (1988), *Forgotten Millions*. London: Paladin.

Cohen D. (1981): *Broadmoor*. Psychology News Press: London.

Cole M. and Maltzmann N. (1968), *Soviet Psychology*. San Francisco: Freeman.

Corson, S. A. (1976), *Psychiatry and Psychology in the USSR*. New York: Plenum.

Digby, A. (1986), *Madness, Medicine and Morality*. Cambridge: Cambridge University Press.

Gostin, L. (1977), *A Human Condition*. London: MIND Publications.

Hill, W. (1985), *Learning: a survey of psychological interpretations*. New York: Harper & Row.

Holland, J. (1976) *A Comparison of American and Soviet Psychiatry* in Corson, S. A. (1976) *op*. cit.

Hoskins, G. (1988) *Reith Lectures*. BBC Publications.

Jordan, N. (1968), *Themes in Speculative Psychology*. London: Tavistock.

Laing, R. D. (1972), *The Politics of Experience*. Harmondsworth: Penguin.

Lauterbach, W. (1985), *Soviet Psychotherapy*. Oxford: Pergamon.

Medvedev, Z. and Medvedev, R. (1971), *A Question of Madness*. London: Macmillan.

Nekipelov (1974), *The Institute of Fools*. A Chronicle of Current Events, No. 42, 1976.

O'Connor, N. (1961), *Recent Soviet Psychology*. Oxford: Pergamon.

(1966) *Recent Soviet Psychology*. Oxford: Pergamon.

Parchomenkow, (1986) *Images of Dissent in the Soviet Union*: Boulder: Praeger.

Pisarev, S. P. (1970), *Soviet Mental Prisons*, Survey, 77, 175–80.

Podrabinek, A. (1980), *Punitive Medicine*. Ann Arbor: Karoma.

Porter, R. (1989), *Anatomy of Madness*. London: Routledge.

Rack, P. (1982) *Race, Culture and Mental Disorders*. London: Tavistock.

Robinson, P. (1989), review of *Dispatches, British Medical Journal*, 21 January 1989.

Scull, A. (1983), *Museums of Madness*. Harmondsworth: Penguin.

Segal, B. (1976), *Involuntary Hospitalisation in the USSR* in Corson, S. A. (ed.) *Psychiatry and Psychology in the USSR*, op. cit.

Seligman, M. (1975), *Helplessness*. San Francisco: *Freeman*.

Sherrington, R., Gurling, H. et al (1988) Localising a gene for schizophrenia, *Nature*, 10 Nov. 1988 p. 164 ff.

Slobin, D. (1966), *Handbook of Soviet Psychology for the XVIIIth International Congress of Psychology in Moscow*. White Plains, N.J.: International Arts and Science Press.

Szasz, T. (1972), *The Manufacture of Madness*. London: Routledge.

Tichonenko, V. (1988) *Moscow Psychiatric Aid Service*. Novosti

Valsiner, J. (1988) *Development Psychology in the USSR*. Brighton: Harvester.

Wing, J. B. (1977), *Reasoning about Madness*. Oxford: Oxford University Press.

Winn, R. B. (1961), *Soviet Psychology: a symposium*. New York: New York Philosophical Library.

Index